Penguin Handbooks
Stammering

Ann Irwin was born in 1924 and brought up in Suffolk. During the war she served in the W.R.N.S., and after that became a student at the Kingdon-Ward School of Speech Therapy in London. Upon qualifying in 1949, she moved to Newcastle-on-Tyne where she worked for three years as assistant to the Chief Speech Therapist at the Royal Victoria Infirmary and other Newcastle hospitals. It was during that time that she found that in the wide range of speech, voice and language disorders her particular interest was in stammering. She was awarded a scholarship and a Fulbright travel grant and went to study at the State University of Iowa in the United States, where research into and treatment of stammering were carried out in depth. She earned an M.A. in Speech Pathology from Iowa and then returned to Newcastle, where she continued to work part-time at the Royal Victoria while raising her own family.

Ann Irwin is currently acting in charge of the Department of Speech Therapy at the Royal Victoria Infirmary.

STAMMERING
Practical Help for All Ages

Ann Irwin

Penguin Books

Penguin Books Ltd, Harmondsworth,
Middlesex, England
Penguin Books, 625 Madison Avenue,
New York, New York 10022, U.S.A.
Penguin Books Australia Ltd, Ringwood,
Victoria, Australia
Penguin Books Canada Ltd, 2801 John Street,
Markham, Ontario, Canada L3R 1B4
Penguin Books (N.Z.) Ltd, 182–190 Wairau Road,
Auckland 10, New Zealand

First published 1980

Copyright © Ann Irwin, 1980
All rights reserved

Made and printed in Great Britain by
Richard Clay (The Chaucer Press) Ltd, Bungay, Suffolk
Set in Linotype Pilgrim

Except in the United States of America, this book is
sold subject to the condition that it shall not, by
way of trade or otherwise, be lent, re-sold, hired out,
or otherwise circulated without the publisher's prior
consent in any form of binding or cover other than
that in which it is published and without a similar
condition including this condition being imposed on
the subsequent purchaser

Contents

Foreword 7
Preface 9

Section One

1 General Introduction   13
2 Definition of the Word 'Stammering'   16
3 How Stammering May Develop   18
4 Some Physical Aspects of Stammering   21
5 Some Psychological Aspects of Stammering   25
6 Causes of Stammering   33
7 Therapies for Stammering   40
8 Dr Johnson and Dr Van Riper:
   Theories and Therapies   45
9 Speech Therapy for Children   51

Section Two

10 Introduction to Easy-Stammering   59
11 Anatomy of the Speech Organs   65
12 Easy-Stammering Therapy   72
13 Some Individual Problems   90
14 Easy-Stammering for Children   100
15 Some Results of Easy-Stammering   106

Section Three

16 Speak for Yourself   115

Suggestions for Study   138

Foreword

Stammering is not a disease, but it is an affliction. It may be no more than a mild interruption to the normal free flow of speech, or it may make communication totally impossible for the sufferer and even ruin his whole life. The cause of stammering or stuttering is not known, though two main theories hold sway. Some believe that the stammer results from hidden psychological trauma which the individual suffered during his early childhood. Others feel there is an organic basis, perhaps due to some underlying lack of development of the speech centres of the brain, or perhaps to some aberration in the timing of neuronal mechanisms underlying speech.

Many of the everyday things which we so readily take for granted are extremely complex when we come to think about them. The development of the human adult from a single cell is perhaps even more complex than landing a man on the moon. The development of speech in that individual is also extraordinarily complex, and yet most people achieve normal fluent speech with hardly a conscious thought to the mechanics involved.

If we do not know the basis for stammering, can we possibly manage to treat it? The answer to this question must be that stammering can be helped, if not totally alleviated, in most people who suffer from the condition. It is for this reason that Mrs Irwin has written this book, to bring knowledge, understanding and help to a group of people who often fail to seek assistance. Stammering is made worse by stress and worry, and the first essential is to teach the sufferer something about what is going on when he gets into difficulties over words. Mrs Irwin's book is intended equally to be read by speech therapists and students, and by members of the lay public, both those who suffer from a stammer and those who have relatives with this condition. It is essentially a personal book, and thereby is very readable. It sets out her personal experience over a number of years of treating a number of patients by the method of 'easy-stammering'. As a result of reading the informative chapters, and following the clearly set out method of teaching oneself to control the stammer, I am sure that many people afflicted with this condition will be greatly benefited.

W. G. Bradley, M.A., B.SC., D.M., M.R.C.P.,
Department of Neurology,
New England Medical Centre,
Boston, Mass.

Preface

My intention is that this should be a simple book. The problem called 'stammering' (or, in the U.S.A., 'stuttering') is already so complicated that I find it impossible to get down to the basic issues of the problem unless I view it as simply as possible.

A great many books and numerous papers have been written about concepts and statistics. These are for the serious student who is interested in the subject, and the emphasis is more on the theory than on the therapy. Winston Churchill once said, 'Personally, I like short words', and I must say that I agree with him.

This book is primarily for speech therapists, students of speech therapy, adults who stammer and want to do something about it, and parents of children who stammer. The first section gives a general background to the problem of stammering, the second describes in detail my therapy, which I call 'easy-stammering', and the third section is devoted to patients who speak for themselves. In this section the initials of patients are given, but initials in other parts of the book are fictitious in case anyone should object to their inclusion.

Whether a speech therapist is helping a patient, or whether a person with a stammer is helping himself, it is essential to have some background knowledge of the problem. You are therefore strongly advised not to 'start on the therapy' before reading the background.

My frequent references to 'people who stammer' rather than to 'stammerers' stems from the belief that people are *not* 'stammerers'; they are *people* who have a stammer. It seems equally wrong, to me, when people are referred to as 'diabetics' or 'spastics'. They are *people* who have a condition known as 'diabetes' or 'spasticity'.

A few years after becoming a speech therapist, I was fortunate enough to spend a year in the U.S.A. as a student under the direction of Dr Wendell Johnson. I was fortunate, too, in visiting Dr Van Riper. After returning to England, with the limited time available for treatment here, it took me many years to work out a therapy which was effective, and I am now quite certain that, in the vast majority of cases, it *is* effective. To me, it has been an exciting journey. I hope that you, the reader, will equally enjoy journeying into the problem of stammering and what we can do about it.

I am extremely grateful to Dr M. E. Morley, D.SC., F.C.S.T., F.A.C.S.T. (Hon.), who has given me much help by reading and correcting the typescript of this book.

Section One

1

General Introduction

He makes His sun rise on the evil and the good,
and sends rain on the just and the unjust.

Matthew 5:45

People usually quote Moses as the first person recorded as having a stammer (Exodus 4:10, 'O Lord, I have never been a man of ready speech, never in my life ... I am slow and hesitant of speech').

Be this as it may, it is certain that people have suffered from the affliction of stammering all through the ages. It has always been with us and, what is more, it is not confined to any one part of the world, or even to many parts. It is world-wide. So when one is trying to deal with stammering, it is as well to remember that the problem is both age-old and universal; there is no quick cure.

People must have tried to cure their own stammers for literally thousands of years; more recently people have tried to cure other people's stammers, but a cure has never been found. During the eighteenth and nineteenth centuries it was believed by some surgeons that stammering was caused by a physical defect of the speech organs. In Britain tonsils were sometimes removed, but in France and Germany operations took place for slitting the tongue or for removing sections of it. These methods were taken up by other surgeons, who presumably wanted to jump on the bandwagon, until it became quite a widespread practice. This was, indeed, a strange happening because these grim operations did not even help the stammering, but it does indicate the lengths to which people would go in the hope of gaining relief from their stammers. Probably due to the shock of the operation, the stammer tended to decrease or disappear for a short while, but it always returned.

It is of great interest, I think, that in England at just about this same period (i.e. 1860) there was a Dr Hunt* who apparently treated stammering with great success, as did his father before him. He taught his patients to 'speak consciously, as other men speak unconsciously'. His treatment is not made known in any detail, as he believed (very understandably) that the secret of success was in the application of the system, and not in the system itself. This doctor was the only light on the horizon at that time, so far as I know, and it came as a revelation to me, when I read a reprint of his book, to discover that well over a hundred years ago somebody had so much insight, good sense, and understanding of the problem of stammering.

Apart from this far-seeing doctor, it is only during the last fifty years or so that real progress has been made in the understanding of the problem and in methods of relieving it. This has largely come about, as I see it, because two determined young men in the U.S.A., separately to begin with, and both with crippling stammers, sought help wherever they could find it. Seek as they might, they did not really find any substantial help anywhere until, finally, they began to help themselves. They learned about themselves and about their own stammering condition, and they worked on it and worked on it, until they achieved fluency or near fluency. Then much later, and with university appointments, they began to teach other people with stammers to help themselves, and to teach students of speech therapy how to help people with stammers. The two men were Dr Charles Van Riper at Western Michigan University, and the late Dr Wendell Johnson at the State University of Iowa.

A great deal of research has been undertaken during the last fifty years in an attempt to fathom the cause (or causes) of stammering and to find an effective method (or methods) of treatment. There are now many theories about the cause, and there are many therapies. Stammering has been treated with

* J. Hunt, *Stammering and Stuttering, Their Nature and Treatment*, originally published 1861; reprint: introduction by E. J. Schaffer, New York, Hafner, 1967.

varying degrees of success, but we still do not know either its cause or its cure. That is not to say that nobody is ever cured; this does happen, but it is more realistic to view a stammer as a problem which exists and which can be greatly improved. The word 'cure' means that the condition has been completely eradicated, in which case it will never appear again, under any conditions. This I believe to be rare, except in children.

Unlike the European surgeons, we know that stammering is in no way associated with defects of the organs of speech. But before we laugh (or cry) at their methods, we might do well to bear in mind that none of us has found a cure, and that to pat ourselves on the back would be a bit premature.

2

Definition of the Word 'Stammering'

> 'Have you guessed the riddle yet?' the Hatter said,
> turning to Alice again.
>   'No, I give it up,' Alice replied: 'What's the answer?'
>   'I haven't the slightest idea,' said the Hatter.
>   'Nor I,' said the March Hare.
>   Alice sighed wearily. 'I think you might do something
> better with the time,' she said, 'than waste it
> asking riddles with no answers.'
>
> Lewis Carroll

If you asked a hundred different people to define the word 'stammering', you would probably get nearly a hundred different answers.

The *Pocket Oxford Dictionary* defines a stammer as 'to speak haltingly, especially with checks at particular sounds', but even this is an inadequate definition, as most non-stammerers speak haltingly at times, and people with stammers who speak with 'checks at particular sounds' do not *always* get checked on those particular sounds.

Adults who stammer have described the condition to me in various ways: 'The words get stuck in my throat', 'I'm unable to push the words out', 'Sometimes I can't talk', 'I'm all right sometimes', 'I have to change words', and even 'I get a pain in my chest' and 'I can't shop'.

Parents of children who stammer also describe the condition in a host of different ways, for example: 'He speaks quicker than he thinks', 'He thinks quicker than he speaks', 'I think he is too sensitive', 'I think it is his nerves', 'He talks too quickly', 'He is too highly strung', and 'He doesn't really stammer, he stutters.'

Definition of the Word 'Stammering' · 17

My point is that people who stammer, and parents of children who stammer, almost invariably describe the condition in *general terms*. After all, when stammers occur, something happens to the organs of speech. The front of the tongue may be stuck to the roof of the mouth, the lips may be pushed hard together and apparently unable to break apart, or the teeth may be clenched together, and so on. But when I ask the question, 'What happens when you stammer?' the answer is almost certain to be in general terms, such as 'Sometimes I can't talk', rather than in specific terms, such as 'My lips get stuck together and I get a tremor of the jaw' or 'I tend to repeat the first sound of some words'. I think that people who stammer are usually so emotionally involved with the fact that they are stammering, that they are unable to take an objective view of it by noticing what is happening to their speech organs during the times that their stammers occur.

Many speech therapists have tried to define the condition but these definitions tend to be either so short, e.g. 'a disorder of speech in which fluency is impaired', that they only *partly* describe what stammering is and are therefore inadequate, or so long that they become cumbersome and unsuitable for everyday use.

3

How Stammering May Develop

Sweet Benjamin, since thou art young,
And hast not yet the use of tongue,
Make it thy slave, while thou art free;
Imprison it, lest it do thee.

John Hoskins

It is normal for children to begin to use their first words from before one year of age until after two years. Their first words are usually heralded with much glee by the parents, as if speaking was one of the most exciting things that could possibly happen in life. Members of the family try to get the little child to repeat his first word again and again, for the sheer joy of hearing it. Then they eagerly await the next word that the child will speak, and the performance is repeated.

It is little wonder that the beginnings of speech are greeted with such joy. The single words are soon joined together to make little phrases; then follow the sentences, and the child can begin to use his speech as his tool, to express whatever he chooses; to find freedom in expression. But what is it, somewhere along the line, which causes a child to stop using his speech fluently, and begin to hesitate more than the average child does? What makes his utterances begin to show signs of tension? Some people might say, for example, that his upbringing is too strict; yet some children begin to stammer when the upbringing is not strict. We just do not know the reason or reasons that a child begins to stammer. But we do know that the stammer, in little children, very frequently disappears so long as it is dealt with in the right way.

Naturally parents usually try to do what they consider best for their child. Therefore, when they see that something in their child's speech is not quite the same as it was before, they begin to take notice of it and, naturally, they sometimes begin to try to correct it. This is the beginning of trouble. If only parents knew that the trouble is not so much in the first signs of tension in some of the words the child speaks, but in the correcting of it, they would probably finish up with a child who does not stammer, instead of one who does.

Let us imagine a child called Timothy. He is four years old. His speech has developed normally, and he has been speaking with full sentences, and as fluently as any other child, for over a year. He is alert and intelligent. He is developing quickly, as young children do; he is experiencing new things every hour of his life. His life is full of surprises because he is learning so much, so quickly. A week ago he could ride his bicycle with stabilizers; yesterday he rode it without stabilizers. Yesterday the lawn was green; today it is white with snow; he has made a snowman and been for a ride on the sledge. His conscious life is busy with his new experiences. But his speech is an unconscious process, he doesn't need to think about that; it just happens. If he had noticed it, but he hasn't, he would have known that all people, and especially young children, hesitate when they talk. This particular day Timothy hesitates a bit more than he usually does, and with a bit of tension. Timothy, of course, doesn't notice but his mother does. Perhaps it was nothing, but perhaps she had better listen carefully tomorrow just to make sure everything is all right. Tomorrow Mother has forgotten all about it, until Timothy happens to show a slight sign of tension on one of his many words. Then she remembers about the tension yesterday. She is just a little anxious but hopes everything will be all right soon. She will be watchful for a few months and see what happens.

Well, after a few months the tension is not only still there, but worse. She feels sure now that he has a stammer. What can she do? Why, try to stop him 'doing it', what else can she do? So when he stammers she begins to say things like 'Take your time', 'Take a deep breath before you speak', or 'What are you talking like that for?' Timothy hadn't realized that he was doing anything different, until she told him about it. Now, when he has little stammers, and Mother makes remarks about it or looks worried, he too is beginning to become aware of them. The more she notices them, the more he notices them, until he begins to try not to 'do it'. The more he tries not to 'do it' the worse it gets. He *must* 'do it' because *it's there*, but he cannot 'do it' because he wants his speech to be acceptable to his parents; he wants their approval. This is the conflict. This is the beginning of a true stammer for Timothy, who may now never experience the pleasures of fluent communication.

Once a stammer is what we might call established, it tends to be self-perpetuating and to go on, over the years, getting worse. The person who stammers almost invariably goes on trying not to 'do it'. Either consciously or subconsciously he struggles against it, and fights it, and resorts to all sorts of tricks to try to beat it. He tries to overcome it by 'doing things' which bring some relief to the stammer, only to find later that the stammer is as bad as ever, and on top of it he now 'does things' while he is stammering.

4

Some Physical Aspects of Stammering

It is hard for thee to kick against the pricks.
                                   Acts of the Apostles 9:5

The most obvious thing, to me, about an established stammer, is its complexity. I sometimes sit in the clinic watching a person stammering, and wonder at so many parts of the body being involved. Getting severely stuck on just one word might involve extreme tension of the lips, larynx, tongue, and jaw, possibly accompanied by closed eyes, clenched hands, twisted feet, and sweat running down the face. Once the word is finally uttered, the patient can probably say it a second time, with no apparent tension anywhere.

Any one person's stammer appears to be different from any other person's stammer; you never really find two alike. One person will stammer on a small percentage of words, another on perhaps as much as 50 per cent. The person who doesn't stammer very much will probably have periods when he stammers quite frequently. The person who stammers on a large percentage of words will probably have periods when he doesn't stammer very much. Some people stammer when they are talking but not when they are reading aloud; others stammer both when speaking and reading. Some people are completely fluent when they talk or read aloud, so long as they are completely alone and nobody can hear them. Others stammer when they are alone, whether they are talking or reading, although the stammer is usually not so severe as when they talk or read to other people. Almost all people with stammers are able to read fluently if several people are reading at the same time, and almost invariably they can sing with no sign of stammering at all.

When stammering first begins in a little child it is usually of a simple repetitive type, e.g. 'Mummy c.c.c.can I go out to play?' and 'Ah.ah.are you coming to kiss me goodnight?' With the growing awareness of his hesitations, from whatever source it may come, and with his increasing attempts not to 'do it', the tensions tend to get greater and the stammer gradually becomes more complex. The simple repetitions begin to show signs of increasing tension, paving the way to complete 'blocks' when no sound is coming out at all, but where the tension is even greater.

People with advanced stammers present some of a vast variety of physical symptoms, which are deviations from normal speech, and which would probably never have become part of the stammer if they had never tried to stop stammering. The following symptoms are typical:

1. Tense (or extremely tense) repetitions of sounds.
2. Tense (or extremely tense) prolongations of sounds.
3. Complete blocks, with voice:
    (a) at the level of the lips (as for 'b');
    (b) with the tip of the tongue behind the upper front teeth (as for 'd');
    (c) with the back of the tongue against the soft palate (as for 'g');
    (d) at the level of the larynx (i.e. vocal cords).
4. Complete blocks, but without voice, at all levels in no. 3 above.
5. Speaking on an in-breath.

Sometimes the position of the speech organs, before a sound is attempted, does not bear any relationship to that sound. For example, for a word beginning with a vowel, like 'America', when the mouth should be slightly open, the person who is stammering may close his lips (as for 'b') and push and push. Again, for a word beginning with a consonant, such as 'potato', when the two lips should be placed together, he might open his mouth wide and tensely pronounce 'ah – ah'.

Added to the basic stammer, there are usually other physical signs of struggle, e.g. sniffing; nasal snorts; licking the lips; tremors of the lips; staring eyes; closing the eyes; poor eye contact (staring at the carpet while stammering); tongue-thrusting to varying degrees; jerking the head, or throwing it backwards or forwards; clenching hands; banging the knee with the hand; twisting the feet; stamping; sweating; unusual breathing patterns.

Usually the stammer is greatest at the beginning of a word and the beginning of a conversation. Frequently it is greatest at the beginning of a sentence.

Dividing sounds into groups

Many of us first learned the vowel sounds – 'a', 'e', 'i', 'o', 'u' – on our five fingers. The remainder of the sounds are consonants, and may be divided into two groups, (1) continuants and (2) plosives. All except six of the consonants are what we call 'continuant' sounds. They are called continuants because we can continue saying them for as long as our breath lasts. If you say f— (not ef), for example, you can go on saying f— until you run out of breath. The same is true of all the other continuant consonants, which are 'v', 'th', 's', 'z', 'sh', 'l', 'w', 'y', 'r', 'm', 'n', and 'h'. Technically, two others, 'ch' and 'j', are not true continuants, but we may class them as such. The remainder of the sounds, the other six, are 'p', 'b', 't', 'd', 'k', and 'g'. These six sounds are called 'plosives'; when producing them we literally have to 'explode' something before the sound is heard. For 'p' and 'b', the lips are together; the sound only comes once the lips are 'exploded' apart. The same principle is true of 't', 'd', 'k', and 'g'. So, with a continuant, sound is coming out all the time we are saying it; with a plosive, the sound only comes after we have released it.

The letter 'c' is not mentioned; 'c' as in 'cat' is identical in sound to 'k' as in 'kitten'; 'c' as in 'city' is identical in sound to 's' as in 'sit'. The letter 'q' is also omitted as its sound is 'k' followed by 'w'.

Stammering on particular sounds

It is rarely that people stammer on only one particular group of sounds, but it is fairly common for stammering to occur much more frequently on one or two groups than on the others. As an aid to analysing the stammer, I divide sounds into five groups:

1. Vowels

2. Consonants $\begin{cases} \text{Plosives} \\ \text{Nasals} \\ \text{Semi-vowels} \\ \text{Remainder} \end{cases}$ all continuants

The nasal sounds are 'm' and 'n'. These are the only two sounds which come through the nose instead of the mouth, (apart from 'ng' as in 'sing', which only comes in the middle of, or at the end of, a word).

The two semi-vowels are 'y' and 'w'. These sounds begin with a vowel and immediately glide on to another vowel sound.

Sometimes stammering is virtually confined to the *plosive* consonants 'p', 'b', 't', 'd', 'k', 'g', or to some of these six consonants. Sometimes a person will stammer far more on the *vowels* than on any other group. Sometimes the *nasal* sounds are particularly troublesome, or the *semi-vowels*, or it may be the nasals *and* the plosives, and so on.

One other very important physical aspect of stammering is the excessive speed at which a person who stammers often talks. I believe that he has taught himself to do this in the hope that he will be able to get to the end of his sentence before the stammer hits him. He hopes in vain. All that happens is that his speech becomes so rapid that it is frequently unintelligible; the words get concertinaed together, whole syllables are omitted and the stammer is still there. As with other attempts to overcome the stammer by doing things about it, the rapid speech then becomes one more addition to the basic stammer, hindering rather than helping.

I trust that I have not given the impression that the symptoms of a stammer may be, for example, 'tense repetitions of plosive consonants, with poor eye-contact and a head-jerk'. There is much more likely to be a wide variety of physical symptoms, but with a *tendency* to stammer in particular ways, and on particular groups of sounds.

5

Some Psychological Aspects of Stammering

The Centipede was happy quite,
Until the Toad in fun
Said 'Pray which leg goes after which?'
And worked her mind to such a pitch,
She lay distracted in the ditch
Considering how to run.

Mrs Edmund Craster

When I ask people how they *feel* when they stammer, they almost always answer either, 'I feel ashamed', or, 'I feel embarrassed.' I have said that stammering is a complex problem, but that is really an understatement. On top of the basic stammer, and other signs of struggle, come all the reactions to stammering.

Each person tackles his stammer, either consciously or unconsciously, in his own way. The adult who stammers has, for years, been trying to overcome it by doing things about it. Usually what he has done has made the stammer worse, and he gets more involved, not only physically, but emotionally, with his speech. He has deep feelings about himself, about his speech, about how he appears to other people and how he is (or is not) going to cope with speaking situations. He lives in a world of uncertainty, never knowing for sure whether or not he is going to make a fool of himself. He feels not only shame and embarrassment but also inadequacy and insecurity. A patient said to me recently, 'You see the trouble is that you never know what to expect. You never know if you'll be able to talk or not. And just when you want to talk really well to somebody, you find that you're quite speechless; you just can't say anything.'

Why can't they talk well, just when they want to? One of

the reasons could be that they are a bit afraid of how the listener might react. This could happen especially when they want to 'talk really well to somebody', that is, when they want to make a good impression, or at least not make a bad impression. People with stammers tend to imagine that listeners are reacting to their stammers when they are *not*, in fact, reacting. I recall Mr C.R., who went into a chemist's shop to buy a toothbrush, and while he was stammering the assistant was gaping at him, open-mouthed. Mr C.R. felt dreadful about that, and little wonder. A few weeks later he had to buy some stamps at the post office. He said to me, 'Everyone in the post office was laughing at me.' I thought it odd that everyone in the post office should, in fact, have laughed, so I said, 'Mr C.R. In what way did they laugh? Did they giggle or laugh aloud, or what?' 'No,' he said, 'they didn't laugh aloud.' 'How then did they laugh, if they didn't laugh aloud?' Mr C.R. concluded, 'They didn't laugh aloud; they didn't make any actual noise, but I knew they were laughing at me because I could *feel* it.'

Now I know that, on some occasions, people do laugh at stammering, but people with stammers frequently make life more difficult for themselves by *imagining* that people are laughing at them or reacting to the stammer in some other unpleasant way. A different example of someone expecting other people to react to his stammer was given to me by Mr N.R. He went to buy some fish and chips. When he got to the shop there was quite a queue, which he joined. More people came and joined the queue, so after waiting for half an hour Mr N.R. was more and more aware of the growing number of people, forming the queue behind him. As he neared the counter, he began to wonder whether he would ever be able to buy the fish and chips. It wasn't the buying of them which worried him; it was all the people behind, who he was sure would be listening to his stammer. By the time he reached the counter he decided he couldn't face 'having all the people staring at him', so he made as if to leave the shop but actually joined the end of the queue, so he had to wait all over again! This time he was last, so he finally managed to get his fish and chips. Strangely, he was not embarrassed by getting as far as the counter and then leaving it to join the back of the queue. I would have expected more people to stare or grin at him for doing this than to have stared or grinned if they had heard him stammering. Mr N.R., however, knew from experience that his stammer would be worse than usual in this particular situation.

Most people with stammers know which are their hardest and which are their easiest speaking situations. It is usually (but not always) when a person is trying not to stammer that he stammers most. A stammer almost always varies in different situations; often the worst situations are: with strangers; at interviews; in a group of people; with people in authority (the doctor, the boss); in shops; on the telephone; buying tickets (theatre, cinema, bus, train, etc.). The easiest speaking situations for a person who stammers are very frequently: with his family; with his friends (both sexes); talking to his juniors.

The stammer will also differ according to the *words used*, and to the *sounds* those words begin with. Usually a stammer occurs more on some sounds than on others, and often people know certain words which they just cannot say. When a person notices that he is stammering badly on a particular word or a particular sound, he begins to fear that he will be unable to say it next time. With this apprehension, he is likely to stammer on it next time, and so he builds up, in his mind, words and sounds that he feels incapable of saying. I remember a patient who told me that he could not say words beginning with 'p'. I noticed that, as he talked, he was in fact saying *some* words beginning with 'p' with no stammer at all. I discussed this with him and asked why he thought he always stammered on words beginning with 'p'. He answered that he had been on the London Underground and tried to buy a ticket to Piccadilly and he had stammered very severely on the word. The fact that he could not say 'Piccadilly' did not mean that he could never say 'p'; it is more likely to have been that buying a ticket was a difficult speaking situation.

As people notice that they stammer on certain words they frequently begin to avoid saying them. I can just imagine the 'Piccadilly' man asking, next time, for Leicester Square, and walking the extra few hundred yards, rather than try to say

'Piccadilly' again. This would be typical. Then, once he has deliberately avoided saying 'Piccadilly' it would be even more difficult to say next time. After he has asked for Leicester Square a dozen times, he has convinced himself that he cannot say 'Piccadilly' because he cannot get out the first 'p'. He may well be able to say 'pickle' with no stammer but he has probably never taken note of the fact.

The more somebody learns to fear certain words, the more he teaches himself to avoid saying them. Sometimes he can avoid saying them altogether (for example, he can hand over the correct amount of money for his bus fare, without saying anything) but much more often it leads to word 'switching'. If he cannot say 'circle' he can say 'round'; if he cannot say 'Monday' he can say 'the day after tomorrow', and so on. A patient recently was unable to refer to his sister as 'my sister', and instead had to say, 'I'm her brother.'

Some people switch words just a little and some do it consistently. Some enjoy doing it because it helps them to stammer less; others hate doing it because it makes them feel inadequate, and also because they often finish up expressing themselves badly, and not saying what they really wanted to say. All people who switch words get really worried when they come to something which is impossible to switch, such as a name and address or a telephone number.

People vary in their desire and ability to switch. I well remember Miss G.T. She was a beautiful young lady of about twenty, and she came from a wealthy family in the United States. Her family gave big parties, and Miss G.T. said to me, 'I can join the party at 8 p.m. and talk until 2 a.m. without *any* stammer at all, but I *never* finish saying what I started out to say. I switch from one topic to another, depending on which words I can use. I always get by, and what I say usually makes sense, but I get *so* frustrated because I want to say so much, and I never say any of it.'

Nearer home was the case of Mr J.G. He was a professional man and determined not to 'make a fool of himself' by stammering. He was in his thirties when I knew him and he had practised the art of switching since he was a little boy. I have never known anyone, before or since I knew him, switch with such excellence. I had hours of conversation with him and he talked fluently all the time. In contrast with Miss G.T., Mr J.G. *did* say everything he set out to say; he always had another word to use. But it didn't really help him; every time he had to switch a word he felt demoralized. He had all the frustration and loss of confidence which one might have expected him to have if he had stammered instead. He hated switching, but could not bring himself to stammer instead, because a lot of his associates did not even know that he had a stammer. When, in the clinical situation, he was persuaded to talk without switching, his stammer was really severe.

These are two somewhat extreme examples, but they illustrate the lengths to which some people will go to talk without stammering, even though the experience brings them a feeling of utter frustration.

Most people who stammer also avoid *situations* if they expect to stammer badly in them. They may avoid just one situation, frequently that of joining in a group conversation, but it is more usual to avoid, or avoid as far as possible, several other situations. The most difficult ones are often: using a telephone, shopping, and buying tickets. School children and students often do not ask questions in class, even if they believe the question is an important one and they want to know the answer. They also avoid answering questions in the classroom if they possibly can.

Mr R.E., a university student, was recently asked to read aloud to a class an essay which he had written. The lecturer was new and was not aware that Mr R.E. had a stammer. Mr R.E. refused. The lecturer insisted that he should read the essay. Mr R.E. again said he would not read it. Then ensued a verbal fight, and both got very angry. Finally another student told the lecturer that Mr R.E. could not read aloud because he stammered severely when reading. The lecturer (very decently, I thought) apologized to Mr R.E. and all was peace again. Although a popular student, Mr R.E. was quite unable to bring himself to tell the lecturer, in front of the class, that he had a stammer; also, he had always managed somehow to avoid reading to the class, because that was a particularly difficult situation for him.

So far, we have seen that people who stammer often avoid words altogether by just not saying them; avoid certain words by switching to other similar words; and avoid situations which are distressing to them. These are only part of the picture of avoidance techniques. They also try to avoid words, by postponing them, although they intend to say them eventually; these are known as 'postponements'. People do a variety of things in order to 'put off' the word they expect to stammer on, before uttering the actual word. These postponements often take the form of repetitions; usually of a word or a phrase. Somebody is, for example, trying to say 'I was in a shop'; he can say 'I was in a' but not 'shop', so he says 'I was in a-a-a-a-a-a' before finally saying 'shop'. In this case, he is repeating a word which is in the sentence he is trying to say. Sometimes he will repeat a word or phrase which is *not* part of his original sentence, for example, 'I was in a I mean I mean I mean shop' or 'I was in a you know you know you know shop.'

A common example of phrase repetition is when a person is trying to say his name. Suppose his name to be John Brown, and he knows he can say 'John' all right, but not 'Brown'. He says, 'My name is John B ... my name is John B ... my name is John B ...'. He cannot get farther than the 'B' because he is stammering on that sound, and he may well repeat the phrase from two or three times to a dozen times or more. He is postponing the word 'Brown' by repeating the phrase preceding it, over and over again. Watching someone doing this reminds me of a horse trying to jump a fence, but, instead of jumping when he reaches it, going back for another try. It doesn't matter how often the horse tries, the fence is not going to disappear; it will still be there for him to jump finally, whether he tries once or a dozen times.

I think that people use postponements because at one time they have been useful. They start as tricks. Say that somebody is, originally, going to stammer and finds that, by saying 'I mean' in front of the troublesome word, he can get it out without any stammer. It works, so he is going to stick to it, and little wonder. But it does not *go on* working. A month or a year later it no longer helps the troublesome words; the aid has worn thin, but by then it is too late to discard it; it has become part of the stammer. In a similar way to the physical tricks (closing eyes, knee banging, etc.) started as an attempt to overcome the stammer, so do people try mental tricks to try to overcome it. Tricks just do not help, except in the short term, and thus the basic stammer gets added to and added to, ending up as an extremely complicated picture of avoidances in whatever forms they may come. The man who said that if people could avoid avoiding they wouldn't stammer must have been a very wise man.

People who stammer vary enormously in their attitude towards stammering. Some of the most obvious complaints are that it is a social barrier; a disadvantage in jobs, often stopping promotion; an embarrassment in many speaking situations; a frustrating disability when it stops people from expressing their feelings or making known their views. Sometimes they get left out of conversations, and often people will not wait for them to speak. Often the listener tries to help by supplying the word he thinks the person with the stammer is trying to say; reaction to this help varies. Some people are only too grateful to have the word said for them (and they can, if they want, usually repeat the troublesome word, without a stammer, once somebody else has said it for them); others are furious at having their word supplied for them, and it is even worse if the wrong word is supplied.

I recall a patient whose attitude to stammering was extreme. She was a very pretty young girl of eighteen and her stammer was what I would describe as slight. Often she did not stammer at all; when she did stammer, it was a 'halt' lasting for only a second or two. She said to me, 'I'd rather have leprosy.' Thinking she was exaggerating to get her point across, I said, 'Now come on, be honest about it. Let us talk about what leprosy involves and then you will see how much better off you are than someone with leprosy.' She repeated that she would rather have leprosy. Fortunately, it is rare for a person who stammers to take such an extreme attitude.

Some writers liken stammering to some of the most crippling ailments; they compare it with blindness, deafness, paralysis, or being in constant pain. Perhaps I should not judge, because I do not stammer, but, for myself, I feel sure that stammering would not be comparable with these crippling ailments.

6

Causes of Stammering

*...but what is it that hath burnt thine heart?
For thy speech flickers like a blown-out flame.*

              Algernon Charles Swinburne

When I have asked adults who stammer, or parents of children who stammer, what they think the cause was, I have been given a huge variety of answers; here are a few of them: 'He broke a thermometer, in his mouth, when he was two'; 'He imitated his father'; 'He copied his friend who stammered'; 'He fell out of his pram'; 'It started with measles'; 'The sofa caught fire'; 'I was knocked down by a car'; 'I got into trouble when I broke a window'; and so on. More frequent than any of these, though, is 'It was when he started school.'

If one questions a parent more thoroughly, it often turns out that the exact onset of stammering cannot be remembered. This is an imaginary but typical conversation:

Q. 'You say Billy began to stammer when the sofa caught fire?'
A. 'Yes, he got an awful shock; he was sitting on it.'
Q. 'Exactly how old was he then?'
A. 'About three.'
Q. 'Yes, but can you remember his *exact* age?'
A. 'It's too long ago, and with three other children I cannot remember the details.'
Q. 'Do you remember Billy's third birthday? Did he have a party?'
A. 'Yes, I remember his third birthday; we gave him a puppy.'
Q. 'Had his stammer already started when you gave him the puppy?'
A. 'No, he was a beautiful talker then.'
Q. 'Did the sofa catch fire before or after Billy had the puppy?'
A. 'Oh, it must have been before he had the puppy. I remember, because the puppy was allowed to sit just on the patched up end of the sofa, so the fire must have come before the puppy.'

Q. 'So, in fact, the stammer must have started *after* Billy's third birthday?'
A. 'Yes, it must.'
Q. 'So it looks as if the sofa catching fire was *not* the cause of the stammer?'
A. 'That's right; but it can't have been long after that before he started stammering.'

In this instance, it was not true that the stammer started when the sofa caught fire. I am not suggesting that this was an impossible reason for a stammer to begin; I am suggesting that parents tend to look for a cause of the stammer quite some time after it has started. They frequently forget dates and details, and tend to look back to anything which gave the child a shock somewhere around the time that the stammer started. Having recalled a shock, they then tend to be satisfied that the shock was the cause of the stammer, even though the timing of the shock and the stammer did not coincide.

Sometimes, however, parents are quite adamant about the cause, and it appears that, in some instances, the stammer did definitely follow, for example, being knocked down by a car or some similar shock. Quite often parents who cannot remember details do appear to remember with certainty that the stammer began within the first few months of starting school.

People within the profession of speech therapy also hold different opinions about the cause of stammering. Millions of words must have been written about it by those who treat it, but we still do not know what the cause, or causes, are. A great deal of research has been carried out, especially in the U.S.A., and this has taught us a lot about what stammering is *not*, but not so much about what *it is*.

The three most popular theories are that the cause of stammering is:
1. A neurosis, or
2. Learned behaviour, or
3. Organic.

1. Neurosis

Much has been written about stammering being a neurosis, especially by psychologists, but it seems that many people make statements about this without being able to substantiate their claims.* Take the following few examples: 'The primary cause of stammering is psychological; fear states prevent the brain from properly controlling the speech organs'; 'Stammering is a symptom of an emotionally disturbed personality. It has its roots in fear or in some deep-seated emotional conflict'; 'Compulsive repetitions occur because of anxiety and guilt'; 'Stammering is a phobia of words'; 'Stammering is a psychological difficulty'; 'Stammering is the great speech neurosis.' These near-quotes are, of course, taken out of context, but nevertheless they are statements which say 'I believe' without giving any proper grounds for the belief.

If stammering is a neurosis, the first question one might ask is: 'Are people who stammer neurotic?' Most research and experience shows that people who stammer are a great deal more anxious about their speech than are people who do not stammer, but that they are otherwise no more neurotic than other people.

2. Learned behaviour

All of us are normally non-fluent to a greater or lesser extent; we all tend to 'um' and 'er' and repeat words and phrases. Children, naturally, learn language haltingly; some more haltingly than others. It is believed by some people that this halting speech persists into later life because the child has learned to stammer through expecting to do so. If a child expects to stammer, a conflict develops because of his desire to speak and his desire to avoid stammering. If he finds that he stammers in certain situations then, when he is in the same situation again, he will expect to respond in the same way, and the stammer

---

*F. H. Hahn, *Stuttering, Significant Theories and Therapies*, 2nd ed. prepared by E. S. Hahn, Stanford, California, Stanford University Press, 1968.

becomes self-perpetuating. It is said that the satisfaction, to the person who stammers, of finally getting the word out, reinforces the stammer and that he goes on stammering to repeat (unconsciously) that satisfaction.

It is further suggested that stammering is a by-product of *emotional* learning. If, for example, a child experiences a strong emotion of fear, this may make it difficult to organize the flow of thought, so that fluent speech becomes impossible. Having experienced stammering when he is very frightened about something, then the next time he is frightened he may respond in the same way, with a stammer. In other words, his behaviour has been learned.

Stammering has often been described as 'a bad habit'. One authority says that the theory of learned behaviour means that stammering is a bad habit, but it does not explain how or why the bad habit began.

3. Organic

This term indicates that the cause of stammering is physical. Nowadays, people who hold this theory usually believe the brain to be, in some way, responsible. In the past, however, all sorts of organs were given the blame.

During the present century there has been much speculation about the central nervous system being responsible, especially in that there may be some irregularity in the integrations of the part of the nervous system required for speech. And at one time it was quite widely believed that stammering was associated with handedness. If a left-handed child was made to become right-handed, this might cause him to stammer. Several studies showed this, apparently, to be the case, but then other questions were posed.* Why did some children *not* stammer when they were made to change from being left-handed to being right-handed? Was it the change of hand which caused the stammer, or was it the emotional difficulties which arose out of

---

*W. Johnson, *Stuttering and What You Can Do About It*, Minneapolis, University of Minnesota Press, 1961.

having to change the hand? Are people truly right- or left-handed, or are they a bit of both? Many questions led on to further research and there have now been something like one hundred studies, over the last fifty years, related to this subject. Much research has shown a similarity in handedness between those who stammer and those who do not, and the prevailing opinion today is that stammering is not caused by change of hand, but the door on this subject does not appear to be entirely closed.

'Predisposition' is sometimes said to be the reason for stammering; in other words, people are born that way, with an inherited tendency. Some children, in times of stress, may turn to such things as nail-biting and thumb-sucking but they do not stammer. Other children, in times of stress, may begin to stammer. Some children, however, begin to stammer when there is no apparent stress. Why? Well, some people say that if a child begins to stammer and there is no conceivable reason why this should have happened, then he must have been predisposed to do so. (The question of inheritance is discussed further on page 47.)

Another organic theory has been that people who stammer may differ, biochemically, from those who do not. Tests have been made to analyse the composition of the blood, and there were suggestions of differences, but further research has indicated this is not so.

For myself, I find it difficult to know what to believe. I cannot accept that stammering is a neurosis, on the basis that I have known so many people who stammer, over so many years, and I just do not find them neurotic. Not a very scientific attitude perhaps, but clinical experience counts for something. The theory of learned behaviour I also find somewhat unconvincing. I am the firmest believer that learned behaviour accounts for the greater part of an established stammer, even up to 99 per cent, but still, I believe a stammer preceded all the behaviour which made the stammer grow.

The theory of predisposition may well be true, but it is an assumption, and it is an easy way out to say 'he was predisposed to stammering'. It would be a great help if we knew that certain people were so predisposed, and if we knew what made them predisposed, but we do not know.

Whilst heeding the probability that there may be more causes than one, I have nevertheless been impressed by the number of mothers who have said to me something like this: 'He used to be a beautiful talker, then he just started stammering.' One minute, it seems, his speech was normal, and then suddenly he stammered. When I have asked these mothers to show me, with their mouths, what happened when the child first stammered, they have demonstrated it for me, showing *tension* of the speech organs. It seems that, in these cases, the stammer just happened. Some mothers have said that the stammer came on gradually but have insisted that neither they nor anybody else corrected it or took any notice of it. Other mothers have agreed, when questioned, that they might have corrected normal non-fluencies.

One could try to argue: 'Stammering *cannot* have an organic basis because, if it did, people would not have periods of fluency.' However, this does not follow, because speech is the responsibility, not just of the lips and tongue, but also of the mind and brain.

Personally, I prefer the organic theory, accepting in the light of present knowledge that there may be some mistiming of impulses within the brain, associated with the circuit shown in the diagram.

I find it quite impossible, however, to separate the physical self from the mental self, and both of these from learned behaviour. They are, as I see it, not only closely associated but inseparable. Somebody's theory is that stammering is a neurosis. Then a psychologist may tell us that a neurosis is caused chemically. Well, if it is chemical, it is organic. And where does learned behaviour come in? Has one learned to be neurotic because of a chemical imbalance or has one's body chemistry learned to become imbalanced because of a state of mind? Let us look at an example of this. I am trying to wash up, fetch somebody from school, and prepare a meal in one hour of time. I need two hours to do these things, so I get a headache. I virtually never get a headache unless I am trying to do things at double the speed they take to do. There must have been a *first time*, under these conditions, when I got a headache. The *following* times could be called learned behaviour, because by then my body had learned to behave in this way. That leaves the cause of the headache to be either in the mind or in the body, if mind and body can be viewed separately.

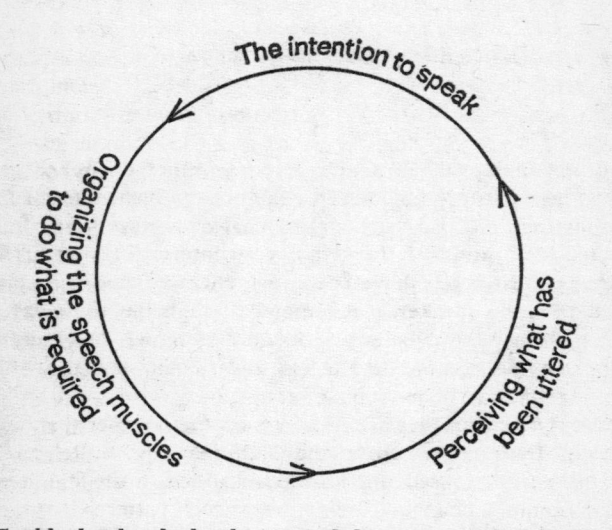

Diagram: a circular flow with three arrows labelled "The intention to speak", "Perceiving what has been uttered", and "Organizing the speech muscles to do what is required".

Could the headache be caused by my *mind*, which was anxious because of the impossibility of doing two hours work in one hour, without my *body chemistry* being equally responsible, in that it brought about the physical changes which produced the headache? Which one was the culprit? Surely neither one was responsible, but rather the way the two acted together.

So, although I favour the organic theory, I believe that the mind cannot be viewed separately from the body. The search for the cause of stammering must go on – it is vitally important from a preventive standpoint; but to the person with an established stammer, it does not matter whether it started in the body, or in the mind, or by learned behaviour, or all three; what matters is its alleviation.

7

Therapies for Stammering

The eagerness of a listener quickens the tongue of a narrator.

Charlotte Brontë

The first therapy I know of is that of Demosthenes (385 B.C.), the Greek orator, who chewed pebbles to prevent himself from stammering. He also used a great deal of gesture when he delivered his orations. I think it is very interesting that his self-therapy must surely have been very effective, because he was such a famous speaker. It is somewhat laughable, these days, to think of chewing pebbles to control a stammer, but I suppose it was a 'distraction device' (as also would be the gesture-making); that is, he must have been so busy working his tongue round the pebbles that his mind was on *them* rather than on his speech. Distractions from the stammer (by more modern means!) are still used, and still found to lessen the stammering – for example, changing the natural speech pattern. If someone with a stammer talks with a foreign accent, or in a sing-song voice, or in any rhythmical way, his stammer is likely to be greatly reduced. Other distractions do not even require the changing of the natural speech pattern; just dancing, for example, or some other rhythmical activity, is enough to reduce stammering.

Over the years, many therapies have been used in the attempt to find an answer to the problem. There have been, and still are, opposing schools of thought about whether one should treat the symptoms or the cause. People who believe that stammering is caused by an emotionally disturbed personality tend to treat it by trying to re-educate that personality, the idea being that, if a maladjusted personality can become adjusted, then the stammer will look after itself. A completely opposite view is that the person with a stammer should be taught the rules of perfect speaking, practising vocal exercises and paying attention to articulation, pitch of voice, and correct breathing. Other therapies were based on 'chewing', and on whispering or sighing, leading on later to voiced speech.

Looking at some of the things that have been said about therapy,* during the last thirty years or so, I wonder why so many people have made an already complex subject more and more complex. Why do they not try to simplify it? In some cases an enormous number of tests and medical checks were required. Anyone might think that the patients were candidates being selected for a journey to the moon instead of being about to embark on a course of speech therapy. Here are some of the requirements: investigations into neurological, psychiatric, psychological, sociological, medical, and nutritional states; ear, nose, and throat examination; physical and mental hygiene; psychotherapy, physiotherapy, and environmental therapy; answering personality questionnaires and writing down attitudes towards family, health, education, sex, religion, politics, etc. Obviously, a patient needs to be in good health to get the most out of any course of treatment, but it does look as if, in an attempt to discover and eliminate all physical and psychological deviations, too many professions were brought in, in order to form a multi-therapy attack.

Hypnotism was used widely at one time; immediate results are often very impressive but unfortunately the effects wear off. This can be very distressing as someone may think he is better, only to find out a few days later that he is as bad as ever. Various drugs have also been tried but did not seem to be much use. Nowadays, however, tranquillizers do seem to be helpful in some cases. I would not personally advocate the use of drugs at all, except in extreme cases of anxiety associated with stammering, and then only for a short period while coping with some very difficult aspect of therapy.

Relaxation used to be a very popular therapy and it is still used, but very much less than it used to be. The patient is

*F. H. Hahn, op. cit.

taught how to relax his body, both lying down and sitting, and it is then possible for him to talk without stammering, or with greatly reduced stammering; the aim of the therapy is to give him the repeated experience of easy speaking. With regular practice of relaxation, the patient learns to become aware of unnecessary tensions and then gradually becomes able to control these.

Years ago, when I used relaxation therapy, I was not impressed by the results I got. Many therapists must have shared this experience because this therapy has now been largely abandoned. A small number of therapists did get very good results, however. I know of one man who was said to have lost his stammer entirely, purely with general relaxation; he didn't even talk to the therapist about himself or his troubles.

Another man got over his stammer completely, by whispering. As a young lad he was not allowed to chat in bed; one night he wanted to tell his brother something and whispered his tale, finding to his astonishment that he did not stammer. He thereupon decided to whisper, and this he did for two years. At the end of the two years he began to talk with voice again, but his stammer had gone.

New techniques have been discovered, more recently, which have been found to reduce stammering. I will give only the briefest outline of these; details can be found in books and speech journals by anyone who wants to know more about them.

One such technique is 'shadowing'. A tape-recording is made of someone else's speech and the patient listens to it through ear-phones; he immediately repeats what he hears, using a quiet voice, so he is virtually listening and speaking at the same time. Sometimes he can repeat what he hears with complete fluency. As with so many therapies, the problem is carrying over into everyday speech the speech which can be achieved in the clinical situation. My own feeling is that this is even more difficult when an 'aid', that is, a piece of equipment, is used, which cannot be used outside the clinic. However, some people have reported a degree of success with this method.

Another technique involves the use of 'delayed auditory feedback' (Daf). Using a magnetic tape-recording it is possible, with a suitable appliance, to return a person's speech back into his ears, through ear-phones, with a delay of about one fifth of a second. This reduces stammering, sometimes dramatically. It is not usually considered to be a complete therapy in itself, but is very useful as a clinical tool. Reports on its value vary, but in many cases it appears that stammering has lessened considerably with the use of Daf. This is an extremely interesting discovery for several reasons. One is that some people, who do not stammer, *do* stammer using the Daf machine. The implication is that stammering appears to be closely associated with the *timing* between speaking and receiving back that speech, when the ear hears. This new knowledge could alter the whole conception of both the cause of stammering and its treatment. How interesting it is to remember that Hippocrates, the Father of Medicine, thought that stammering was due, in part, to an 'affection of the ears'. One assumed him to mean that he associated it with some sort of hearing trouble, but who knows whether he was thinking more in terms of auditory feedback?

'Syllable-timed-speech' is a therapy which has become quite widely used in England over the last few years. With this, the patient learns to give the same amount of time and the same amount of stress to each syllable. For example 'My name is Jonathan Brown' would become 'My name is Jon a than Brown'. It sounds rather unnatural, but on the other hand it is fairly easy to learn. Some people can make their speech sound more natural after much practice. There are indications that syllable-timed-speech is more effectively learned when therapy is given intensively, e.g. full time for a fortnight, rather than on a half-hour-per-week basis. Some people claim that this therapy is very helpful indeed when it is combined with other forms of help.

The use of the 'electronic metronome' is another technique which has been tried with considerable success. The patient wears an ear-piece which gives a 'tick' in his ear; the speed of the tick can be adjusted. He has to learn to match the natural stress in his speech with the tick. For example, if you say 'I had a lovely walk along the beach today', you will notice that the words 'lovely' and 'beach' are the words which stand out: they are the stressed words. So, those two words must match with the tick of the metronome. The patient learns, with graded exercises, how to use the metronome effectively. A lot of this work is done at home and he does not need such regular help as with other therapies. One very interesting aspect of this therapy is that there is no personal relationship between the patient and the therapist. With all the therapies I know of, except this one, the personal relationship between patient and therapist is of supreme importance, but here it is virtually non-existent. The patient is given the metronome and the exercises, and is taught how to carry them out; then he goes and gets on with it.

'Masking' is another method used in the treatment of stammering; to be effective, speech must be completely masked, which means that the speaker must not be able to hear his own speech. The Edinburgh Masker is a quite recently developed electronic device which has received much publicity. The speaker wears a small microphone on his throat and, when he speaks, noise is transmitted into both ears. This device is only for the use of adults and is intended only to be used if conventional therapy has failed. In a few cases it has a dramatic effect on the stammer, to the extent that the speaker is completely fluent. Other people get no help from it, or only a very little. The majority of those who wish to have a masker find a very considerable improvement when wearing it. The advantages of the Edinburgh Masker are that the speaker has to make no effort to improve his stammer and that, to whatever extent it helps him, the improvement is immediate. The disadvantages are: having to wear the microphone, ear moulds with flexes, and control box (which is small); never hearing oneself speak when using it; having a loud noise in one's ears whenever speaking; and finding no lasting improvement in the stammer once the device is removed. It is not yet known what the long-term benefits might be.

It is impossible to include all the therapies for stammering, because individual therapists work in individual ways, and one just does not know what techniques are employed nor what results are obtained; for this reason, I have only been able to mention the major therapies, other than those which follow in the next chapter.

8

Dr Johnson and Dr Van Riper: Theories and Therapies

Two Voices are there; one is of the Sea,
One of the Mountains; each a mighty voice:
In both ... rejoice.

William Wordsworth

I am determined that this book shall be kept simple and readable. For this reason I have expressly avoided direct quotes, and names of people; if these were included, it would be necessary to give a bibliography, which would immediately give it an 'academic' quality. But two names are so important in the story of stammering that to leave them out would be, to me, like writing a book on Royalty without mentioning the King and Queen. They are the two Americans mentioned in Chapter 1, both professors of speech pathology in university departments, namely, (the late) Wendell Johnson and Charles Van Riper.

When they have given, say, forty to fifty years of their lives to the study and treatment of stammering, and after the vast amount they have contributed in the way of books and research, it would be foolish of me to try to jot down in a few pages what their beliefs are. Let me, instead, try to select some outstanding features, as I see them, which today probably form the basis of the greater part of therapy for people who stammer, especially in the U.S.A.

Wendell Johnson theory

We have already mentioned the hesitations in speech, which everybody has; these are called 'normal non-fluencies'. Children tend to be more non-fluent than adults, and if these hesitations are noticed by anyone, usually the mother, and the child is made *aware* of them, he may develop a stammer. That is, a child who has no stammer becomes conscious of the fact that he is hesitating, and he tries not to hesitate because it brings disapproval. However, he cannot help hesitating, because it is *normal*. The disapproval may take many forms. It could be verbal: the child is told to stop hesitating, to talk slowly, etc. Or it could just be that the mother looks away or looks anxious while the child is being non-fluent. Children are very sensitive to atmosphere, and will sense it quickly if they are not acceptable as they are.

In Wendell Johnson's admirable words, 'The stammer begins not in the mouth of the child, but in the ear of the parent.' Having once diagnosed her child as a stammerer, the mother's behaviour to him changes a little. She begins to act slightly differently towards him, and to say different things. She may sometimes look anxious when he talks; she may tell him to take his time. *Her* behaviour affects the child, so *he* begins to behave slightly differently. He tries not to hesitate; this makes him hesitate more; the greater hesitation worries the mother even more; her anxiety gets across to the child. So grows the vicious circle which makes the normal non-fluencies of childhood begin to show signs of tension and the tension go on increasing.

One can see, here, how the behaviour is learned. But the great thing that Johnson gives us, as against the 'stammering is learned behaviour' school, is a *cause* as well. Please do not confuse Johnson's theory with my imaginary case of Timothy, who began to hesitate *with* tension.

Johnson therapy

Johnson defined stammering as 'an anticipatory, apprehensive, hypertonic, avoidance reaction'. *Fear* is the real heart of the problem. A stammer is built up by fear of words, fear of particular sounds, and fear of certain situations. When you fear, you begin to *avoid* the words, sounds, and situations *which* you fear. You learn to try to avoid stammering. So, to gain control of the stammer, you must stop avoiding. If you stop trying to avoid stammering, you begin to speak normally; or, in one of his typical phrases, 'you must avoid avoiding'.

'Doing the feared thing helps to overcome the fear.' You fear stammering, so learn exactly how you stammer and then go and stammer on purpose. First, stammer in front of a mirror until you know exactly what it is that you do when you stammer; then learn to imitate it; then go and stammer deliberately. This voluntary stammering is NOT for gaining control, but an exercise in throwing caution to the winds. Stop being cautious; go ahead and stammer and the fear of stammering will begin to lessen.

Do not think of stammering as something that *happens* to you. Instead, describe to yourself in real terms everything you DO when you stammer, e.g. 'I am forcing my lips together', 'I am pushing my tongue hard against my palate.' Then say to yourself: 'It is not *happening* to me. I AM DOING IT. WHY am I doing it? Stop pushing so much. I don't *need* to push that hard.'

Do not think of yourself as a stammerer. Learn to handle speaking situations without apologizing for the stammer; and *refuse* to be handicapped. If you do these things, the stammer, which is characterized by hurry and tension, will finally become simple and easy.

Answering the question 'Is stammering hereditary?', Johnson's view was that it certainly runs in families, not because of heredity but because parents who stammer (or who have once had a stammer) will be on the look-out for any signs of stammer in their children, and will correct their normal non-fluencies, thus causing stammers to occur.

He tells a wonderful story[*] about a large family in Iowa, of which, over three generations, several members stammered. Finally, one branch of the family moved to Kansas and they lost touch with the Iowa branch. Two generations later it was discovered that nobody stammered in the Kansas branch, but in Iowa eight out of twenty-four children had stammers, or had previously stammered. In the Iowa branch there was one

[*] Johnson, op. cit.

extremely dominant member of the family, who was regarded as 'chief of the family tribe'. He had very definite views about stammering, and believed it was hereditary and that it should be corrected. His attitude towards stammering, added to his influence over all members of the family, was enough to make the stammering continue in generation after generation. The fifth generation of the Iowa branch, however, sought advice about the problem, and learned to change the previous family attitude towards the speech of their own children. They did not correct the non-fluencies in speech development, and in the sixth generation not one of the forty-four children was regarded as having a stammer.

How fascinating it is that these two important forerunners in the study and treatment of stammering, Johnson and Van Riper, had differing views both on the cause of stammering and on the treatment. Johnson believed that the cause of stammering was *not* organic. His main therapy was directed, not at breaking up the stammer symptoms, but at gaining control of the stammer by 'learning to stop avoiding stammering' and by the advice: 'Don't be so perfectionist and cautious; go ahead and stammer.'

Van Riper theory

The basic cause of the stammer, according to Van Riper, is organic; he suggests that there is a 'disorder of timing' within the brain, causing a disruption of the programming of muscular movements required for speech. He says the precision in timing, which is required by the relevant parts of the brain and speech muscles, is essential to fluent speech. If that timing is not perfect, then a distorted word is produced. On top of the basic stammer come all the forms of 'learned behaviour', which we have already discussed, and which convert (as it were) a snowflake into a snowball.

Van Riper therapy

Any therapy, to be successful, must concentrate on breaking up the contortions and forcings which characterize the stammer;

this deliberate modification of stammering behaviour is based on analysis and understanding. My favourite description of his therapy is, as he put it so appropriately in two words, 'fluent stammering'. The old, tense stammer must be replaced by a smooth and simple pattern of stammering which is free of struggle, avoidance behaviour, and gimmicks.

There are three opportunities on any stammered word to control that stammer; that is, before, during, or after the word. People have a tendency to begin to tense the muscles of speech *before* they actually begin to say something, as if they are preparing themselves to stammer. They are, in other words, 'set to stammer' and this condition he called 'the preparatory set'. The person with the stammer must learn a *new* preparatory set with his speech organs in a state of rest, allowing the first sound of the word to glide into the next sound. Becoming aware of the tension which is present, before speech actually begins, gives the opportunity of modifying that tension.

If the person cannot manage to control the stammer by changing his preparatory set, there is a second chance to control it, after the stammered word has actually commenced, by the use of a 'pull-out'. Here, the patient learns to become aware of the tension which is present when he 'blocks', but, instead of pushing on with the word, he 'pulls out' of the tension and finishes the word with a prolonged, gliding control.

If the block is not successfully controlled by a pull-out, there is a third opportunity to control the stammered word. This is by 'cancellation'. Having completed the stammered word without control, the patient should realize that he has 'pushed' the word out, and then 'cancel' his failure to control at all by repeating the word in an easier way.

The object is not to try to talk without stammering, but to stammer with a change for the better. By using the preparatory set or pull-out or cancellation, the patient is always getting the better of the stammer; he is learning to control the stammer instead of being controlled by it. Every time he succeeds in doing this, he becomes the winner and the stammer becomes the loser; the greater the control, the less the stammer.

Sometimes it is easiest to start with the technique of cancellation; this is comparatively easy to do and, once it is mastered, it is easier to learn pull-outs. Then, when the technique of pull-outs has been mastered, it is easier to learn the technique of changing the preparatory set.

With the use of these three techniques, one is not only learning to control the stammer but also learning a healthier attitude; instead of trying to avoid stammering one is learning that every time a stammer occurs there is an opportunity to get the better of it. If a whole day should pass without a single stammer one would learn nothing; but if hundreds of words have been stammered on, and control has been attempted, then a great deal has been learned.

Van Riper's therapy appears to be almost entirely directed to control of the stammer symptoms, either directly by modifying the symptoms, or indirectly by a change of attitude towards them. He takes a wide view of the angles from which the stammer should be attacked. The person with the stammer must learn to understand both the stammer *and* himself. He must be willing to stammer openly and without embarrassment until the stammer is sufficiently improved not to cause embarrassment. Understanding the stammer will include analysing it by listening to it on a tape recorder and watching it in a mirror, and making notes of everything observed. The patient must also observe the speech of other people who stammer, and be able to describe it. He must read about stammering, to discover what causes have been suggested, and what therapies are in current use. He must carry out many assignments to try to put into practice all the things he has learned, which will enable him to stammer in a more fluent way. He must learn insight into his own behaviour, reactions, and attitudes in general, as well as insight into his stammering behaviour.

Van Riper believes that once a stammer is fully developed the original cause is no longer significant, and that the person should be taught a way of stammering which is sufficiently free of tension to bring no social penalties.

9

Speech Therapy for Children

Always behave as if nothing has happened, no matter what has happened.

Arnold Bennett

Treatment is quite clear cut for children before the school-starting age of five, or almost five. The parents and all members of the family, and all people with whom the child associates (often grannies, aunts, uncles and friends of the parents), must learn not to react to the stammer in any way whatsoever. I say 'learn' because one cannot stop behaving in the way one usually does, without a lot of thought and self-discipline. Whatever people 'do' when the child stammers, they must learn to 'undo'. If you say such things as 'Take your time', 'Take a deep breath', or in any way bring the child's attention to his stammer, then this must be stopped. Then again, if you *do* stop correcting him, that is not enough until you learn to stop looking anxious about it. If you look anxious or make him feel in any way that his speech is unacceptable, you are going to make him try to avoid stammering. It has been pointed out, over and over again, in this book, that almost all of a stammer is built up out of trying to avoid it. Once the child knows that he is free to stammer, then the pressure is off. Once the pressure is off, he can stop avoiding and the tensions will begin to decrease, and gradually the stammer will improve. But to be effective this treatment must include *all* the people who have been reacting to his stammer. It is no good everybody in the immediate family doing the right things if granny or a neighbour is still making the child aware of his stammer.

Don't be in a hurry for the stammer to improve; don't keep counting the weeks or months. It will probably take quite a long time to stop feeling anxious about it, but the sooner the better. Remember, the best thing you can possibly do is to *stop reacting*. If you feel that you need support at this difficult time, I would advise you to go and have a few talks with a speech therapist. It may be wisest to go either alone or with your husband or wife; if the child goes with you he may become aware that all the conversation is about the way he talks.

There are many other things which you can do to help him. Encourage him to talk as much as you possibly can, especially in the situations which do not cause him stress; talk about all the things which interest *him*. Be very patient whilst he is talking, and don't interrupt him, so that he knows he has plenty of time, and does not feel in a hurry to get the words out. The more you talk together, the more he will feel that he matters. This will give him confidence, especially now that he is not being corrected or interrupted. You will find your relationship with him growing closer. If you find your conversation runs low, take the next opportunity to do one of his favourite things (go for a bus ride, a game in the park, or a picnic, possibly) so that he can talk about that with you. Failing this, you could read illustrated story books together and watch his favourite television shows together. I am not suggesting for a moment that you should spoil him; on the contrary, his security will depend on the discipline he has always had. But I am suggesting that he gets every encouragement to talk and that his talking is always welcome; this can be very difficult with a large family and a lot to do, but it is possible to change habits, and it will pay dividends.

Try to avoid situations which cause him stress. If, for example, he finds it especially difficult to talk in front of a group of people, then do not try to get him to talk in that situation. Other situations may cause him stress even when speech is not involved; he may, for example, be frightened of sleeping in the dark or something like that. It will help much more to leave the landing light on than to have a fuss about it; try not to subject him to any unnecessary stresses.

Encourage him to shine at anything he is already good at. Give him every opportunity to grow better and better at these things. If his speech is not so good as other people's, then let him show that he can be good at other things. Anything and everything to improve his confidence.

Send him to bed happy and relaxed; perhaps a game or a story or just a friendly chat will suit him – and a big hug.

Sometimes, when stammering is severe, a child will begin to cry, and may say, 'I can't talk.' I have known this to occur in a child as young as two. He needs reassurance but this is not easy to supply when he is anxious. With a very young child who shows real anxiety about being unable to speak, it is probably wise to distract his attention by saying something like, 'You can tell me about that later', and then take him into a situation in which he is usually fairly fluent, such as playing his favourite game or reading a book of nursery rhymes. Your physical closeness during times of anxiety will help to give him security, whether he is sitting on your knee, holding your hand, or just in the same room as yourself.

When older children say, 'I can't talk', it is preferable to face the fact and answer, for example, 'I think you will be able to say that word if you say it like this'; then demonstrate the easy-stammer for him, in the manner described in Chapter 14, Easy-Stammering for Children.

After your child starts school the situation is slightly different from that of the pre-school child. All that I have said holds good after he begins school, but now you are not able to control his environment so completely. You cannot be sure how the school staff and children are going to behave. So, before he starts school, I suggest that you go along and have a talk with the headteacher and the prospective class teacher. You should tell them that your child has a stammer and that you have been advised that the best thing to do is to ignore it; tell them what I have been telling you about not reacting to it, and why. They should try to ensure that the other school children, also, take no notice of it. It is really impracticable to suggest that he can be kept free of all situations which are stressful, because I am sure it is impossible to go through school without a great many stresses. But, so far as his speech is concerned, the teachers could try to ensure that he is not subjected to unnecessary situations which cause him stress. Having to say his name when the register is called, for example, may be difficult for him and is easily avoidable. Reading aloud may be difficult for him in front of the class; in this case, the teacher may be willing to hear his reading, alone with the child, after the lesson.

Going to school for the first time frequently causes a child to stammer more than usual, until he settles down. When he comes home he will probably be excited, either because he has enjoyed it or because he has hated it. This is a time when parents really need to be patient; listening to everything he says, however long it takes, and then either sharing his enthusiasm or sorting out his problems. Most little children, these days, seem to enjoy school and, with the cooperation of the teachers, there is no reason why a child who has a stammer should not enjoy school as much as anybody else. There is a tendency for stammering to be worse than usual at the beginning of every term, but this may only last a few days.

There is no way of telling how many children 'grow out' of stammering, because these are the ones we don't see. I only know that many mothers come to the clinic and say, 'The doctor said he'd grow out of it', whereas in fact the child has 'grown into' it. This is very disturbing because it is harder, and sometimes impossible, to get over an established stammer than it is to get over a stammer in its early stages. If your concern for your child's speech is great enough to warrant a visit to your doctor for advice, then you should certainly also visit a speech therapist, who will be able to advise you.

Stammering is estimated to affect about 1 per cent of the population. That is quite a substantial percentage. Estimates vary throughout the world but, overall, about one person in every hundred is afflicted in this way. You may have noticed that I refer to people who stammer as 'he' rather than 'she'. This is because about four males to every one female stammer. Again, estimates vary throughout the world; some studies show that eight males to every one female stammer. But, wherever it may be, more males stammer than do females.

Most children appear to be really troubled by their stammer; they know that they speak differently from other people. It is

Speech Therapy for Children · 55

usually like this, but not always. Some children seem to be quite unaware of it; others, just occasionally, know that they have a stammer but it does not seem to bother them at all. For those who are unaware of or untroubled by the stammer, it is probably best to accept it for the time being and seek help, at a later stage, if the stammer persists. Formal 'treatment' is useless if the child is not prepared to cooperate.

Therapy for older children and adults varies in method. For myself, I teach 'easy-stammering' to both children and adults, and this will be explained in Section 2.

Section Two

10

Introduction to Easy-Stammering

Order and simplification are the first steps toward the mastery of a subject.

Thomas Mann

I cannot help being enthusiastic about my therapy of 'easy-stammering'. It is not a new phrase; other people talk about easy-stammering, meaning that one aspect of a total therapy is learning to stammer, by various means, in a less tense manner. My meaning is that the entire therapy is devoted to stammering in an easy way; that is, without tension.

It is very difficult to measure stammering and also to measure stammer improvement. If I make a tape recording of a patient on his first visit to me and later count what percentage of words he stammered on when both speaking and reading, that will tell me just two things. It will tell me what percentage of words he stammered on when he was talking and when he was reading, in one particular situation. It does not tell me how much he stammered ten minutes before he met me, nor how much he will stammer ten minutes after he has left me. Because I am a stranger to him, he will probably stammer more than usual with me; on the other hand, he may be one of those rare people who hardly stammer in the presence of a stranger. My tape recording is not going to tell me how much he stammers with his wife, or his friends, or his boss, or when he is on the telephone, or shopping, or even talking to his dog. He is very likely to stammer not only in various degrees in all these different situations, but his stammer will probably vary according to how he is feeling. He may be tired or depressed, or he may feel full of the joys of spring, and these feelings will affect his speech. My tape recording may tell me that, on his first visit, the patient stammered on 20 per cent of the words. If I take another recording on his second visit he may only stammer on 10 per cent of the words. Does that tell me that he is already much improved, or does it tell me that I am not so much a stranger now and that therefore he stammers much less when he talks to me?

When I first see a patient I make a preliminary list of the things which he does and the things which he avoids when he stammers; the list may run, for example:

symptoms of stammer – severe voiceless blocks; severe repetition of sounds; 'machine-gun' at larynx level; plosives most difficult

switches words frequently
eye-contact poor
avoids talking to groups
will not use telephone
avoids talking to strangers unless essential
says 'you know' a great deal

stammer – best with family and friends; worst with strangers and people in authority, e.g. doctor, boss

I make such a list because it is important for both the patient and myself to know what he does when he stammers, and also because it is very encouraging a few months later to go through the list together, checking on the parts of the stammer which have now been either eliminated or improved. I also sometimes make a tape recording so that we can listen to it weeks or months later, and the patient can make his own assessment of his improvement and, hopefully, say the words which are music to my ears, 'Was I really as bad as that? I can hardly believe it.'

Measuring improvement is also very difficult for the person with the stammer, who usually thinks in terms of 'it's improving'. To help him enlarge on this I tell him about the four measurements I learned in Iowa, which are: Are the stammers less *frequent*? (Do you have fewer of them?); Are the stammers less *severe*? (Is there less tension?); Is their *duration* less? (Are they shorter?); Has your attitude towards stammering improved? (e.g. Do you feel less anxious about it? Are you less embarrassed?) I find this a very helpful thing to do as many people who think their stammers are less tense, for example, do not realize that they are also shorter and occurring less often.

I have given my reasons for not trying to measure stammering accurately in the clinic. I prefer patients to decide for themselves what degree of improvement they have achieved, because it is only they who know. It is quite possible to be virtually stammer-free in the clinic and at home, and to have an overall improvement, and yet still experience situations where the stammer can be quite severe. Apart from one study, which will be discussed later, I have never tried to measure either stammering or its improvement. But I know that almost all my patients improve a great deal as they frequently reckon that 70 to 80 per cent of the stammer has gone; almost always with adults a remnant of the stammer remains. This remainder has to be controlled, and people vary in their ability to do this successfully. Usually it is controlled to the extent that it is not very obvious; sometimes the control is so excellent that the stammer is not noticed at all by the listeners.

I was very impressed by the therapy I saw in the U.S.A. when I was there in 1953, but what I saw was confined to treatment within a university set-up. This was a very different proposition from treatment in England. There, in the U.S.A., the patients were usually students who frequently studied speech therapy, or at least took the courses on stammering. Others came from long distances for weeks of intensive therapy, often working for twelve hours daily on their speech, in one way or another. There seemed to be plenty of time for treatment, several hours a day perhaps; certainly several hours per week.

Back in England, over a period of time, I tried to evaluate the situation as I saw it. I knew of no therapy which was really effective apart from relaxation, and that was only effective in the hands of a few exceptional therapists. Other methods may have provided a way to communicate without stammer, but at the expense of sounding natural. Those did not satisfy me. I could not even contemplate the methods I had seen in the U.S.A. because they were so time-consuming. Just one thing made a permanent impression on me; it was listening to Dr Van Riper talking for hours on end with no stammer at all. Then he told me that he had been stammering all the time but was controlling it. When I heard that, it re-shaped all my previous thinking about therapy; I now knew that it was possible to control a stammer so well that the listener would not hear it. This knowledge would be my starting point.

I knew that the only answer, for me, was to work out a therapy which would try to teach perfect control of the stammer symptoms; at the same time, it would also have to be taught in a matter of hours. Having a home and young family, I was not able to work many sessions at the hospital clinic, and only one session in the evening was to be devoted to adults with stammers. So I had three hours per week for, maybe, ten patients and always other people waiting to start. I decided that I would give two or three separate hours to each patient, followed by several half hours of individual treatment, and after that it would have to be group work, even though it meant just a few minutes for each patient. The question was what to do in that time. I knew what my goal was. I knew that it was unrealistic to hope for cures, that is absolute cures, but I knew now that it was possible to have a stammer which 'didn't show'; that was my goal. It took me many years to work out the details of therapy.

First, I thought, the therapy I wanted had to be simple. Working in a hospital means that you take on everyone who is referred; there is no screening which would enable you to select for treatment just the people who would be most likely to benefit, due to intelligence and other factors.

Second, I believed that I could do without all the paper-work of long and detailed case-histories, autobiographies, attitudes and fears tests, and personality inventories. In fact, it dawned upon me that other people's personalities were not my business. Patients were coming to me for help with stammering, not to discuss their personalities (unless they wanted to). What was more, I thought, so long as the stammers improved, one might expect the fears and attitudes to improve automatically. So I made up my mind to work only on the *symptoms* of stammer-

Introduction to Easy-Stammering · 63

ing, and just ask a *few* questions about fears in so far as they related to the stammer, such as feared speaking situations. I decided, too, always to listen when patients wanted to talk about themselves and their problems, and be prepared to discuss these. As it turns out, they rarely talk about anything which is not related to their stammer.

Third, I tried to look at the problem of stammering, as I saw it, to find out what it is that the patient needs to do in order to master it. One thing he needs to do is to approach his problem quite differently from the way he has been doing; he has always tried to *avoid* stammering, and we know this causes nothing but trouble, so he must revise his attitude and become willing to stammer. This is a complete switch round: after years of trying not to stammer, he must now stammer *deliberately*; but, instead of stammering in the old, tense way, he must learn to stammer with as little tension as possible. Another essential is that the patient should learn to control his stammer instead of being controlled by it. Almost always the person who stammers is completely at the mercy of his stammer; it dictates the time and the place, the degree of severity and which words shall be stammered on. That needs to be changed. The basic stammer may well remain, but at least the patient should be able to learn to dictate his terms to it, that is, that the stammer should be at the mercy of the patient.

These, then, were my basic essentials for therapy:

It must be simple.

It must be taught in a short time.

Speech must sound natural.

There must be two complete reversals in the approach to coping with the stammer, i.e. (1) the patient must learn to be willing to stammer instead of trying to avoid it, but it must be an easy pattern of stammering so that he is willing to do this, and (2) he must learn to control the stammer instead of being controlled by it.

From these basics grew the therapy of easy-stammering which will be explained in Chapter 12.

I want to make two things quite clear. One is that not all of my thinking is original. As one goes through life, learning about stammering from reading, lectures, and conversation, certain things make a permanent impression on one's mind. I suppose I have learned most of what I know from other people, and this has made it possible for me to produce a particular therapy. There is a well-known saying, 'A symphony is greater than the sum of its parts'; many of the parts have been offered to me, in one way or another, but the symphony I believe to be mine.

Second, I claim that I get very good results, and this is so. However, I do not get very good results with everybody. Some patients see me once and never appear again. Some come a few times only. Others return, time and again, saying they forgot to work on their speech or that they didn't have time. Some have such a low intelligence that they are unable to carry out even simple instructions. Some people stop attending when they have improved their stammer sufficiently not to feel embarrassed by it; it no longer worries them although the stammer is still quite in evidence. I cannot help the people who do not attend or who are not prepared to cooperate and work on mastering their stammer. The people who get really good results are the ones who come regularly and work on their speech.

11

Anatomy of the Speech Organs

Suit the action to the word, the word to the action.

William Shakespeare

In the clinic it is not necessary to go into any details of anatomy, as a general rule. One can quickly point to parts of the organs of speech to get across one's meaning. To understand my therapy from the written word, however, it is best to know some simple anatomy, so that what I say can easily be understood. Again, my intention is to keep it as simple as possible and to avoid any unnecessary detail. Naturally, nothing will be gained by reading this chapter if you are already familiar with its contents.

The air which we breathe is the same air with which we speak. Our lungs expand automatically, drawing air into them; it is then expelled from the lungs and, if we are talking at the time, that air is used for speech. On its way out, the air passes through the larynx, which is in the throat, and within the larynx are the vocal cords (at the level of the Adam's apple). The vocal cords (which you can think of as two lips, which may be either closed or apart) are apart when we breathe, so that there is a freeway for the air to go in and out. When we hold our breath the cords are together, in which case the air is held beneath them. When we talk the vocal cords vibrate, and this produces voice.

If you say two similar words, such as 'pan' and 'ban', you will notice that, although they are similar, there is a difference. Again, if you say 'fan' and 'van', you will notice the difference. That is because some sounds are *unvoiced* and others are *voiced*; when the vocal cords are not vibrating, the sound has no voice; when they are vibrating, the sound has voice. Thus the difference between 'pan' and 'ban': 'p' has no voice but 'b' has; other than that the two sounds are identical. The same is true of 'fan' and 'van': 'f' has no voice but 'v' has; other than that, these two sounds are identical. All of the vowel sounds have voice; some of the consonants have voice and some have not. These will be discussed later. (If you were to notice that you can whisper and still differentiate between voiced and unvoiced sounds, I would say yes, you are correct, but a discussion of whispering is not relevant here.)

We now have, then, a stream of air to speak with, which has come up from the lungs and passed through the vocal cords; these have added voice to any sound which requires it, according to what is being spoken (you will see that this is a very rapid process). The formation of sounds, which we call articulation, is determined by various positions of the speech organs. The main organs are the tongue, jaw, lips, teeth, hard palate, soft palate, and nose. You will notice that when you say 'ah' your mouth is open quite wide and your tongue is low in your mouth; when, on the other hand, you say 'ee' your mouth is open just a little bit, your tongue is high in your mouth, and your lips are spread. If you alter the position of your lips you will get a different sound; push them forward from 'ee' and out comes 'oo'. That is how it is with all the sounds of speech; each one requires particular positions of the organs of speech.

The pharynx must also be mentioned, as it plays an important part in speech; this is the space at the very back of the mouth behind the tongue. A diagram (see opposite) may help to clarify what the organs of speech are and where they are.

I find that patients are usually quite unaware of what happens to the organs of speech when talking is in progress; I therefore recommend you to face yourself in a mirror and become familiar with what movements occur in the making of speech sounds. Say 'ah' followed by 'ee' and you will see how the jaw opens and then closes. Say 'p' and 'b' to realize how your lips are used. Say 'm—' and listen to the sound coming out of your nose instead of out of your mouth. Bite your lip, then say a long 'f—' and you will see that, with your top teeth on

Anatomy of the Speech Organs · 67

your lower lip, you get the voiceless 'f'. Put the tip of your tongue behind your top teeth (called the teeth ridge) and say 't'. Say the four vowels 'ah', 'ay', 'ee' and 'oo' and watch how greatly your tongue moves.

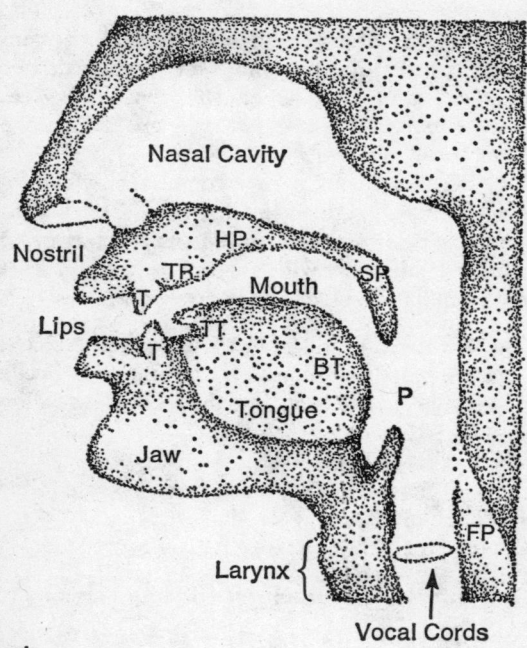

- **T** Teeth
- **HP** Hard Palate
- **SP** Soft Palate
- **TT** Tip of Tongue
- **BT** Back of Tongue
- **P** Pharynx
- **FP** Food Pipe
- **TR** Teeth Ridge

VOWELS

All the vowels are voiced. As with the continuant consonants, mentioned in Chapter 4, we can continue saying the vowel sounds, there being no obstruction in the way.

CONSONANTS

The position of the speech organs varies for all the remaining sounds, which are consonants, and these are best described individually. They are given phonetically, that is, the letters indicate how we *sound* them, not how we *name* them, e.g. p = 'p', not 'pee'; m = 'm', not 'em'.

First we will take the six *plosive* consonants, where obstruction occurs, as was described in Chapter 4. You will see that they go in pairs, being identical apart from whether or not they are voiced. Remember that with the six plosive sounds there is a temporary complete blocking of the flow of air.

- p – the lips are together followed by separation (voiceless).
- b – the lips are together followed by separation (voiced).
- t – the tip of the tongue is against the teeth ridge followed by separation (voiceless).
- d – the same as for 't' but voiced.
- k – the back of the tongue is against the soft palate followed by separation (voiceless).
- g – the same as for 'k' but voiced.

Next we will take the *continuant* consonants; many of these also go in pairs.

- f – the top teeth are on the bottom lip (voiceless).
- v – the same as for 'f' but voiced.
- th – (as in thumb) the tip of the tongue is held between the upper and the lower teeth (voiceless).
- th – (as in that) the same as for 'th' as in thumb but voiced.
- s – the tip of the tongue is behind the bottom teeth; the teeth are together and the lips are slightly spread (voiceless).
- z – the same as for 's' but voiced.
- ch – the tip of the tongue is up as for 't'; the lips are rounded and the teeth together (voiceless).

Anatomy of the Speech Organs · 69

j – the same as for 'ch' but voiced.

sh – the teeth are together and the lips rounded; the front of the tongue is quite high in the mouth (voiceless).

l – the tip of the tongue is against the teeth ridge, air escaping along the sides of the tongue (voiced).

r – the teeth are slightly apart and the tip of the tongue is raised up and curled slightly backwards (voiced). However, many people pronounce this sound differently, e.g. as 'w', or with the top teeth on the lower lip.

h – air from the lungs passes between the vocal cords (voiceless).

There are two consonants which are called *semi-vowels*, being made up of a vowel sound which is quickly followed by another vowel sound:

w – the teeth are slightly apart and the lips rounded for the first part of the sound, i.e. 'oo', which is followed by another vowel, depending on what the word is, e.g. 'what' = 'oo-ot' and 'white' = 'oo-ite' (voiced).

y – the teeth are slightly apart and the lips are well spread for 'ee' which forms the first part of this sound; what follows depends on the word being used, e.g. 'yes' = 'ee-es' and 'yonder' = 'ee-onder' (voiced).

The last two consonants are 'm' and 'n'. These are called *nasal* because, instead of coming through the mouth as do all the other sounds of speech, these two come through the nose.

m – the lips are together, just as they are for 'p' and 'b', but the sound comes through the nose (voiced).

n – the tip of the tongue is up behind the top teeth, against the teeth ridge, exactly the same as for the plosives 't' and 'd', but the sound comes through the nose (voiced).

It is important to understand how the sound 'm' is different, anatomically, from the sounds 'p' and 'b', and how the sound 'n' is different from 't' and 'd'.

The front part of the palate is bony and is therefore called hard; the back part of the palate has no bone and is called soft.

70 · *Stammering*

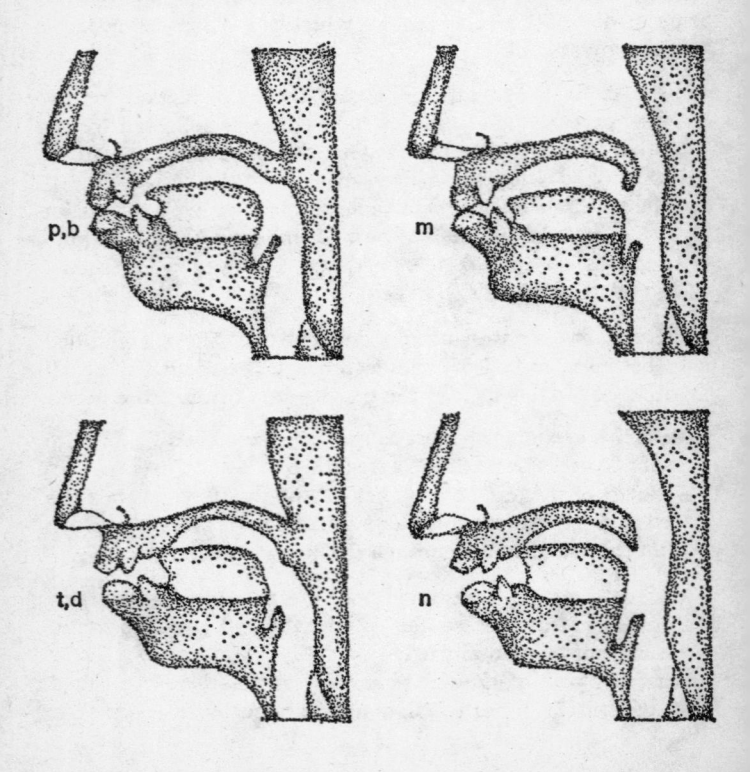

If you open your mouth, in front of a mirror, and say 'ah' you will see that the soft palate rises up; it is very mobile (the little bit that hangs down is called the uvula and is a small part of the soft palate). For all of speech, excepting the nasal sounds, the soft palate rises up in the pharynx and touches the wall at the back of the throat; in so doing, it closes off the passage to the nose so that the sound is forced to come through the mouth. For the nasal sounds, however, the soft palate is down, so that the sound comes through the nose. It *has* to come through the nose because for 'm' and 'n' the mouth is sealed off. When the sound 'm' is made, the lips are together, preventing sound from coming through the mouth, and when the sound 'n' is made the tip of the tongue is against the teeth ridge and this forces the air through the nose. The four diagrams opposite will make this easily understood, and conclude this brief outline of the anatomy of the speech organs.

If you, the reader, have a stammer I feel sure that after studying this chapter you will already have gained just a little bit of confidence. Instead of stammering and having little idea of what is happening to you physically, you can now begin to think in terms of jaw and tongue and teeth and lips and teeth ridge and nose. You can begin to think about the possibility of controlling them, when you stammer.

12

Easy-Stammering Therapy

Wisely and slow; they stumble that run fast.

William Shakespeare

Whenever stammering occurs there is always muscular tension in one or more of the organs of speech; the tension may be in the lips, tongue, jaw, nose, soft palate, pharynx, or larynx, or a mixture of these. To gain control of the stammer you must gain control of the tension by replacing it with muscular ease.

There are two absolute essentials in therapy. One is that you should be well *motivated*, that is, you must really want to learn to control your stammer and not be half-hearted about it. The other is that you can learn to *concentrate* when you are talking, because when you are easy-stammering you have to concentrate not only on what you are saying but also on the way you are saying it. This is very difficult to do because speech is an automatic thing and we don't normally have to think about the way we are talking. It is possible, however; with practice, people learn to concentrate. I warn you, right at the beginning, that learning to control your stammer is very hard work; there is no magic formula or easy way out. You just have to decide whether or not you are prepared to work on your speech; the people who work hard always get a great deal of improvement.

Remember that most of your speech is normal; you don't stammer on every word. Probably 80 per cent of it is normal, in which case it is only 20 per cent we need to work on. We want to get to a situation where the bulk of the stammer has gone and where the remainder is so well controlled that other people don't hear it, or at least don't hear enough of it to take any notice.

The therapy goes in two stages; the first stage is learning

Easy-Stammering Therapy · 73

how to stammer without tension (that is easy-stammering); at this stage, speech does not sound entirely natural. This is the hardest part to learn. The second stage is making the easy-stammer nearer and nearer to normal speech until it sounds completely natural.

The basic principle of easy-stammering is extremely simple. It is this. If you lengthen the *first syllable* of a word sufficiently, it is almost always possible either to say it, or to learn to say it, without tension (i.e. without stammer). A syllable is *one* unit of pronunciation; the word 'new' for example has one syllable, 'newborn' has two syllables, and 'Newcastle' has three syllables.

Please read, and then re-read, this sentence: 'If you lengthen the first syllable of a stammered word sufficiently, it is almost always possible to say that word without tension.' Some people can do this straight away; others have to learn to do it with practice. Let me give you a couple of examples, so that you get the idea. Take the word 'lemon'; make the 'l' and the 'e' both take much more time than they usually do, so that you say a drawled out 'l..e..'; do this two or three times and, after that, add the end of the word at a normal speed, so you will be saying 'l..e..mon'. Say it that way several times to get the feeling of stretching out the first syllable. Now do the same thing with the word 'window'; very slowly now: 'w..i..ndow'. Say it several times; if you are doing it slowly enough, the first sound will be 'oo' so that it becomes 'oo..i..ndow'. That is the basis of easy-stammering, and before we go on to more details I would like you to practise the easy-stammer on a few words. These may well be words that you do not stammer on anyway but that doesn't matter; it is the *idea* you need to practise to start with. Try these:

'f..a..t' (fat),
'th..u..mb' (thumb),
'h..o..spital' (hospital),
's..e..cret' (secret),
'sh..oe..lace' (shoelace),
'ch..e..rry' (cherry),
'j..a..m' (jam),

'y..e..llow' (yellow),
'r..a..bbit' (rabbit),
'm..a..d' (mad),
'n..a..tural' (natural),
'A..m..erica' (America),
'e..v..eryone' (everyone).

You may have noticed that all the words in the above list begin with continuant consonants; I have deliberately missed out words beginning with plosive cononants ('p','b','t','d','k','g') for the moment, as these have to be tackled in a different way. Before explaining what to do with the plosives, I want you to do two things. First, just in case you ever stammer in the middle of words, you should practise an easy-stammer on the second syllable. Doing this is exactly the same as for the first syllable, excepting that the easy-stammer comes in the middle of the word, e.g. 'Atlantic' becomes 'Atl..a..ntic' and 'selfish' becomes 'self..i..sh'.

Second, I want you to practise an easy-stammer on a few words that you frequently stammer on (but not words beginning with plosives) – perhaps your name or the word 'stammer'. 'Stammer' would become 's..ta..mmer', 'John' would become 'J..o..hn', and so on. If you can manage to do this, go on saying them a few times. If you find it difficult to do, then try to easy-stammer on some other words. If you *are* having trouble it is probably because you are hurrying, in which case slow down and try again. It is not possible to say how long the easy-stammer should last because individuals differ; it should last as long as it takes to say the stammered word without tension, perhaps one or two seconds or more.

In these very early stages of treatment the easy-stammer does sound (and it *should* sound) artificially slow. But it doesn't matter; I would suggest that you should not easy-stammer so slowly unless you are on your own or with your family or friends who will know what you are doing and will be trying to help you. To get the idea of easy-stammering it is essential to do it slowly, otherwise the tension does not go. Just a few months ago I had a new patient whose Christian name is

William. During our first therapy session I asked him to say his name; he tried but his name just would not come out, and he gave up. He told me that he had not been able to say his name for more than twenty years; then I asked him how long it would take to say his name if he went on trying and he said, 'About five minutes.' A few minutes later, when we had stopped talking about his name, I asked him to say 'ill' with an easy-stammer ('i..ll..'). He did it perfectly; next I asked him to repeat 'will' after me ('w..i..ll..') and that was perfect too. He did it two or three times. Then I got him to repeat 'W..i..lliam' and he managed that too, with no tension at all. He could hardly believe it and went on and on saying it with an easy-stammer. Since that evening he has always been able to say his name without stammering; the first few weeks he said it with an easy-stammer but after that he found that he did not have to easy-stammer on it, because he did not stammer on it any more.

There are four words with which I want you to become completely familiar, so that you don't have to stop to think what they mean:

1. *Continuant.* This, you will remember, refers to every consonant *except* 'p', 'b', 't', 'd', 'k', 'g'. Strictly, the word 'continuant' refers only to consonant sounds, but for our purposes you should also regard the *vowel* sounds as continuants.
2. *Plosive.* These six sounds are 'p', 'b', 't', 'd', 'k', and 'g'. You must be able to recognize them at once, so they have to be learned.
3. *Fake.* This means deliberately saying a word with an easy-stammer when you do *not* have a true stammer on that word; you are 'faking' an easy-stammer.
4. *Convert.* This means that you are changing a word which you are stammering on (or going to stammer on) into an easy-stammered word; in other words, you are converting a true stammer to an easy-stammer.

If you have carried out the suggestions so far, you will already have the idea of how to easy-stammer on words which begin with continuants. Easy-stammering on the plosives is sometimes much more difficult, so don't get anxious if you find that these take a good deal more practice before you can get them either free of tension or largely free of tension.

Easy-stammering on the plosives

We have to deal with the plosives in a slightly different way from the continuants. Try to lengthen the first syllable of a word beginning with a plosive, e.g. 'baby', and you can see at once that it is an impossibility because you cannot lengthen plosives. There is a complete 'blockage' with these sounds and therefore they cannot be stretched out. So that you really understand that these sounds cannot be lengthened, I would like you to say the following six words, either feeling very carefully what is happening to your lips and tongue, or looking at yourself in a mirror: 'pie', 'boy', 'table', 'door', 'kitten', 'going'.

In order to easy-stammer on a plosive, you have to do two things:
1. It has to be pronounced as *gently* as possible. Put your lips together and say 'p' normally; next, let your lips just touch each other and say 'p' again; there must be no pushing or pressure between the two lips. Then do the same with 'b'. Next, say 't' and 'd' normally; then say them so gently that you can only just feel the tip of your tongue against your teeth ridge. Next, do the same with 'k' and 'g'; first say the sounds normally, then very gently. You should just be able to feel the back of your tongue against the palate. Fortunately the quality of voice is made by the vowel sounds, so saying the plosives in this gentle manner is not going to be noticeable in speech.
2. The remainder of the first syllable is easy-stammered on in the usual way, but if you get a true stammer on the plosive consonant, at the beginning of the word, you must try to concentrate 100 per cent on the remainder of the first syllable in order to get your mind off the plosive.

We will now take the list of six words beginning with plosives, and I want you to say each one with an easy-stammer in the manner I have described. Remember to keep the words sounding completely natural; the only difference one should be able to hear is a lengthening of the vowel sound which follows the gentle plosive. Do not get a break between the plosive and the vowel; for example, with 'pie' the gentle 'p' should *glide* onto the lengthened 'ie' and not be made as a separate sound. Remember, also, to cancel out your normal pronunciation of the plosive and replace it with a very gentle one:

'pie' = (gentle) 'p' and lengthened 'ie';
'boy' = (gentle) 'b' and lengthened 'oy';
'table' = (gentle) 't', lengthened 'a', and normal 'ble';
'door' = (gentle) 'd' and lengthened 'oor';
'kitten' = (gentle) 'k', lengthened 'i', and normal 'tten';
'going' = (gentle) 'g', lengthened 'o', and normal 'ing'.

I find, in the clinic, that the idea of saying the plosives gently is best explained by writing them like this:

'pƤIE..', 'bƁOY..', 'tƮA..BLE', 'dƊOOR..', 'kⱩI..TTEN', 'gƓO..ING'.

I hope that you now know, at least in theory, how to cope with plosives. If, however, you are unable to do them because you are getting true stammers on them (and the plosives do often give a great deal of trouble) there is another way to attempt them. Do exactly as I have already described (i.e. the gentle plosives and lengthening of vowels) but start at the end of the word and work backwards like this:

'ie', 'pie';
'oy', 'boy';
'le', 'able', 'table';
'oor', 'door';
'en', 'itten', 'kitten';
'ing', 'oing', 'going'.

Plosives followed by another consonant

In some words, such as 'pray', two consonants come together before the vowel sound. To easy-stammer on these you do not lengthen the 'r' as that would make the word sound unnatural. Still lengthen the 'ay' and still make a gentle 'p' but, for these words, treat the first two consonants (in this case 'pr') as *one* unit, which will give you a gentle 'pr'. Say some of these for practice:

'pray' = (gentle) 'pr' and lengthened 'ay';
'green' = (gentle) 'gr' and lengthened 'een';
'bluebell' = (gentle) 'bl', lengthened 'ue', and normal 'bell';
'glowing' = (gentle) 'gl', lengthened 'ow', and normal 'ing'.

If you ever stammer on plosive sounds in the *middle* of words, these should be easy-stammered on at the point where the stammer begins, e.g. 'em*b*arrass' (stammer beginning on the 'b') becomes normal 'em', followed by gentle 'b', lengthened 'a', and normal 'rrass'; 'en*c*ounter' becomes normal 'en', followed by gentle 'c', lengthened 'ou', and normal 'nter'.

Some people may question where a first syllable ends and a second syllable begins. In a word like 'blue-bell' it is obvious but what about a word such as 'commonplace'? Is it to be 'comm-on-place' or 'co-mmon-place'? For easy-stammering, the latter is most helpful. To easy-stammer just on the 'co' sounds quite natural, but if the 'm' is also lengthened the result is less natural. Ideally the 'm' should serve as a semi-lengthened link between the 'co' and the normal speed of 'onplace'; being briefer than 'co' but longer than 'onplace' the 'm' then makes the easy-stammer less noticeable. A golden rule, if in doubt, is *always* to easy-stammer on the first *two* sounds or more; never fewer.

The easy-stammer always includes a VOWEL sound.

Speed of speech

We are now nearly ready to start work, but before we do I have to say something about the speed of speech. Many people who stammer talk much more quickly than average; after years of trying to get to the end of a sentence, this is not to be wondered at. The result is, however, that hurried speech increases the stammer; I must have known hundreds of people who stammer, who learn to slow down their speech and then say that the stammer has improved a great deal, even though they have not done anything else to help it. If you are a fast talker you will have to slow speech down if you are going to use the easy-stammer effectively. I am not asking you to talk particularly slowly but only to speak at a reasonable speed. You may or you may not already know if you speak too quickly. If you do, then probably people will frequently ask you what you say. If you are not sure, you should ask your family and friends, or you could time yourself in a situation where you are fluent and count how many words you say in one minute. Anything between 120 and 140 words a minute is reasonable, but if you speak at 180 words per minute remember that that is three words per second, and is certainly too fast for you to concentrate not only on what you are saying but also on how you are saying it. If you believe that you need to slow down, you are the only person who can do it. Other people can help if you ask them to remind you when you talk too quickly – they can help you but they cannot speak slower for you; you have to remember to do this yourself. It is helpful to practise both speaking and reading *very* slowly when you are quite alone; this helps you to both *feel* and *listen* to yourself talking slowly. Later, when you are talking with other people you should be able to catch yourself out if you find yourself speaking rapidly, in which case you must, of course, slow down. Do not start on easy-stammering until you are talking at a reasonable speed because there will be no chance of success.

Stage one in easy-stammering

I believe that nothing succeeds like success, so I want you to take one step at a time, and really work at that one thing until you are successful. There is no given time for each stage in therapy but a week should be the absolute minimum for any stage. Some may take weeks or even months of conscientious practice.

First you have to teach yourself what easy-stammering is – what it feels like and what it sounds like. To do this, you take a newspaper with narrow columns, shut yourself in a room where nobody can hear you, and practise *faking* easy-stammers from this reading material; of course, you must read *aloud*.

It is almost certain that you will have no, or very few, true stammers in this situation, so it is quite easy to fake easy-stammers. You know now that this means you have to lengthen the first syllable of the words you are easy-stammering on. I want you deliberately to easy-stammer on the *first syllable* of the *first word* of *every line* from columns in a newspaper, and to do this *every day* for not less than a week. Practise for at least half an hour daily, but not for more than an hour. Remember it is always the first syllable you practise on; in the word 'around' the easy-stammer begins on the 'a' not on the 'r'.

I will take a passage, underlining the syllables you easy-stammer on to make sure you know what to do. For this, and for whatever practice you do, always approach your work gently and *never rush anything*.

<u>Des</u>pite his advantages it is
<u>quite</u> clear that he minimizes
<u>ra</u>ther than exaggerates his internal
<u>strug</u>gle to keep himself fit, mentally
<u>and</u> physically, to face the world when
<u>the</u> hour should come for his release.
<u>Those</u> who saw his first press
<u>con</u>ferences on television know how
<u>well</u> he succeeded. Certainly from
<u>a</u> course of self-examination and
<u>his</u> study of assorted literature has
<u>been</u> born a writer of great quality.
<u>The</u> wry humour that keeps appearing
<u>is</u> remarkable.

I hope, when you faked easy-stammers on that passage, that you were aware of which words began with plosives, and that you coped with them in the correct way. After a few days of practice you may find that easy-stammer faking when reading is easy to do, but you need to go on with it; it is a very valuable exercise because you are teaching your brain what easy-stammering is. Reading may soon come easily but using easy-stammering in speech is much more difficult and your brain is then going to have to react much more quickly. So let the idea of easy-stammer sink in to your brain so that, when the time comes, it will know what you are trying to do.

Stage two

Stage two is precisely the same as stage one, except that this time you do your easy-stammer reading practice in the presence of a member of your family or a friend. Choose someone to whom you are close, and tell him or her what easy-stammering is so that he or she knows what you are trying to do and can tell you if you are getting any tension on the words you are trying to easy-stammer on.

As you are now reading in front of someone else you may well get some true stammers; don't take any notice of these because at the moment you are only working on *faking* easy-stammers on the first syllable of every line of your newspaper. If you take your time you will probably find that you can fake the easy-stammers with your friend listening, but if you *do* get true stammers on the words you are trying to easy-stammer on, try again with increased lengthening of those particular syllables. If the plosives give particular trouble in this situation, you should work on those words in the way I have already described, i.e. ic-fic-ific-rific-errific-t/e..rrific.

Stage three

Now I want you to begin *converting* true stammers into easy ones. It is best to practise this in reading before you attempt to use it in speech. If possible, practise in front of the same friend. Stop faking on the first syllable; just begin to read and really concentrate so that you notice the true stammers. Go slowly. As soon as you feel (or hear) a stammer begin, stop and pause for a second before attempting that word with an easy-stammer, then drag out the first syllable of that word in exactly the same way as you did when faking the easy-stammers. Don't get disheartened if you find this difficult or even impossible to do at first. Keep on practising until you get some success with it; once you have got some success you will get more and more successes if you keep on trying, and if you know exactly what it is you are trying to do. If converting stammers from reading proves to be difficult at first, it is probably because you are reading and/or easy-stammering too quickly.

Once you feel that you are making real progress with converting true stammers to easy ones, in front of someone else, you should vary this practice by both faking *and* converting in some of your practice sessions. Keep to your newspapers and choose a different column every time. You will fake an easy-stammer on the first syllable of the line and then, if you get a true stammer along that line, you will stop and convert any true stammer to an easy one. Always STOP and pause a second when a true stammer begins. When you stammer your muscles are in a state of tension; they cannot go from a state of tension into a state of ease without a break, so it is absolutely essential that you pause at this point. The pause also gives you a chance to collect your wits and decide how to easy-stammer on the troublesome word.

It is impossible to help with every particular problem without a personal conversation to find out what those particular problems are. Some readers with stammers may find that everything is going beautifully so far; others may be wondering how to cope with a particular aspect of their stammer at this point. If you feel that you need the help and support of a speech therapist, I would strongly advise you to go to one. Ask your doctor or your local hospital how to be put in touch with one. The speech therapist may or may not be familiar with easy-stammering therapy but she or he will be able to give you help with your particular problems. You might even go through the whole therapy, as given in this book, with the therapist if you feel it would be more satisfactory to have support. Working with somebody who understands speech problems could make your task much easier.

Before we move on to stage four I must tell you that it is somewhat rare for people to be 100 per cent successful in converting their true stammers to easy ones when reading to a friend, as early in therapy as this. Keep working at it, but so long as you believe that you now know what easy-stammering is and what it *feels* like to stammer without tension, and so long as you have produced literally hundreds of converted stammers (without *any* tension) when you were reading, you are ready to move on to stage four. If you do not happen to stammer at all when reading you will, of course, have missed out on this practice and will have to begin converting stammers in speech instead of in reading.

There are three things I need to point out before embarking on the important stage four. One is that, as you make progress, you will discover things about your stammer. You will almost certainly find that some sounds give more difficulty than others do; you will also become more aware of the things that you 'do' when you stammer. Naturally, when you are dealing with a problem it is necessary to know what the problem is; if plosives give you the most trouble, it is obviously helpful to know this so that you can be on the look-out for plosives, in order to deal with them. Similarly, if the most obvious aspect of your stammer is, for example, a tongue thrust, then you will be more able to deal with it effectively if you are aware of it. But, although you should be aware of what you do when you stammer, I do not want you to be concentrating on these things when you are easy-stammering; your entire concentration should be on easy-stammering in the way I have told you. This means that you have only one thing to concentrate on; if you can get a perfect easy-stammer then you cannot, by definition, get any tension. Thus in therapy we find that all other signs of stammering disappear so long as the easy-stammer is truly easy. There is no need to try *not* to do things; if you hit your knee with your hand, get a pain in your chest, throw back your head, thrust out your tongue, close your eyes tightly, start off a word with a lot of noise which should not be there, or anything else, these things do not matter. If you can manage to do just one thing, easy-stammering, you will find that all other signs of stammer automatically go.

Secondly, usually people do not know in advance all the words they are going to stammer on, in which case it is necessary to *stop* when the stammer begins and then attempt, after a brief pause, an easy-stammer. Most people know *some* of the words they are going to stammer on; in this case you should always fake an easy-stammer on that word *before* the true stammer begins. If you are going to say your name, for example, 'Philip', and you know you stammer when you say your name, then do not wait for the tension to start but say 'Ph..i..lip' which will probably enable you to say it with no tension at all.

Thirdly, when you begin to use easy-stammering in speech it is essential to do it in an organized way. Do not wait until you are in a mess and then try to switch on the easy-stammer; this doesn't give it a chance. You must decide in *advance* in which situation you are going to easy-stammer; then as you enter that situation you must remember what you are going to do, and having entered that situation you must concentrate on the easy-stammer.

Stage four

Continue with your daily reading practice, both faking and converting.

Now you should begin using easy-stammers in your speech – that is, converting the true stammers to easy ones. It is very important that you give yourself a chance to succeed when you do this; every time you succeed you will gain just a little bit of confidence and I believe that confidence is more help than anything else.

You should first decide with whom you are going to easy-stammer and, if possible, tell those people what you are going to do. Start with the people closest to you, preferably your family as you will be with them a great deal of the time. Next, decide what situations you are going to easy-stammer in; you cannot do it all the time at first, so you should choose, perhaps, meal times or entire evenings. For the sake of brevity, let us suppose that you have chosen to practise with your wife at all meal times; tell her what you have decided and ask her to help you remember to do it at every meal, and after each meal to discuss your performance with you. She must be aware that, even though you are concentrating hard on easy-stammering, it is an art that has to be learned and is not going to be successful every time you try to apply it. I do not care for a great deal of interruption during conversation, so it is better for her just to say, 'Oy', to remind you that you are not easy-stammering, than to keep saying to you, 'You didn't easy-stammer on that word.'

If you happen to stammer quite a lot with your wife, you will get in a lot of practice in converting true stammers to easy ones during the course of a week; if you only stammer a little in the first situation you have chosen for converting your stammers, then you should *fake* easy-stammers in your conversations so that you get in plenty of practice.

Once you feel that you are capable of converting your stammers fairly successfully with the person or people with whom you started, then you should increase the time that you attempt to easy-stammer with them. If your practice is at home and you are out at work most of the day, then try to easy-stammer *all* the time you are at home. If your practice has been with your friends, then try to easy-stammer *all* the time you are with them. You should have the intention to easy-stammer, in your mind, before you enter any situation in which you are going to use it; if at times you forget about it, then your true stammer should act as a reminder to use the easy-stammer. Keeping your sentences short and uncomplicated will be very helpful to you in these early stages. Remember this!

Your practice, in this stage, may cover a period of two weeks or longer. When you feel that you are really beginning to control your stammer, instead of being controlled by it, you are ready to extend the situations in which you will easy-stammer.

Stage five

Keep on with your daily reading, both faking and converting.

First, write down a list of the speaking situations you go into (and also situations you avoid); then list them in such a way that the easiest situation, where you stammer least, heads the list, the next easiest situation comes second, and so on, so that the hardest situation is at the bottom. I am going to make up a list and then explain how to apply easy-stammering for this particular list (you, of course, will have to follow your own list):

home,
girl friend,
other friends,
work,
shopping,
strangers,
buying tickets (avoid, if possible),
telephone (avoid altogether).

The easy-stammer is probably very good at home by now, after all the practice, and you may find that you have fewer stammers than you used to in that situation. Now, little by little, we have to increase the situations where easy-stammering is used (occasionally, somebody is capable of using easy-stammer in almost all situations once he has mastered it in one situation, but he should do this only if the easy-stammer is successful in all situations; otherwise it causes confusion). Our object is finally to reach the bottom of the list and be able to easy-stammer in that situation. You do not get an automatic 'carry-over' into other situations. Your easy-stammer at home could be 100 per cent but this does not mean that you will be able to easy-stammer in shops or with your boss. (Although there is no automatic carry-over of easy-stammering into other situations, extreme signs of struggle, such as squeaking in the throat, speaking on an in-breath, or tongue-thrusting, will frequently disappear in the difficult situations, once they have been eliminated in the easy situations.) You will have to work on easy-stammering in each situation before you gain success in it. Any one situation may have to be sub-divided into several situations; I have one patient, at the moment, who has divided his complicated business life into twelve separate situations.

There is a big gulf between easy-stammering at home and easy-stammering on the telephone, and I think of all the stages in between the two as 'bridge-building'. To build the bridge you must work through your list, one situation at a time, until you can convert true stammers to easy ones in that situation, more or less all the time. Do not expect 100 per cent success in any situation, but let that be your aim.

Keep everything as simple and as calm as you can. Each

situation has to be tackled in the same way; you are now going to begin easy-stammering with your girl friend. You meet her, you have easy-stammering in your mind, you have only one thing to concentrate on in speech and that, of course, is easy-stammering. Tell her all about it so that she knows exactly what you are trying to do and so that she can help you. Every time you are with her you should try to easy-stammer on every word on which you expect to stammer and on every word on which you begin to stammer. Keep up your easy-stammer at home during this time and, when you can also manage it with your girl friend, you begin, in exactly the same way, with all your other friends.

Try not to lose any ground you have gained; once you are doing well with your family and with your girl friend, you must keep up your speech concentration with them as well as beginning to easy-stammer in the next situation, which is with all your friends. This is not so difficult as it may appear, because once you are controlling your speech well in any situation, you will find that you stammer less in that particular situation. If you continue to control well you will find that the easy-stammer becomes more and more automatic.

Continued easy-stammer reading practice is always helpful, for as long as you are working on your speech, but once you are easy-stammering well in most situations it is sufficient if you reduce the reading time to five or ten minutes daily.

Continue through your list, concentrating in one situation after another on the easy-stammer. You will probably find that it comes more easily to you in some situations than in others; this is to be expected. Do not push yourself to the extent that you feel anxious about it, as anxiety will do anything but help you. Imagine, for example, that you have worked your way through easy-stammering at work, when shopping, and with strangers and you now have only two situations left, namely, buying tickets and talking on the telephone, the two situations which you have avoided. Don't feel that you *must* now start trying to easy-stammer in those situations; wait until you have got enough confidence to attempt them and can look upon them as a challenge rather than a worry. I am reminded of a patient

I have at present who had not used a telephone at all for five years. One evening he came in grinning from ear to ear and said, 'I've got some good news for you; since I was here last week I have made two telephone calls.' Suddenly he had felt confident enough to treat his old fear as a challenge; there was no pressure but rather an attitude of adventure.

We will deal in the next chapter with individual problems which may have arisen but, for the moment, let us suppose that things have gone well for you and that you are now at the point where you are easy-stammering excellently in some situations, and very well in most others. If this is so, the bulk of your stammer will have disappeared, and your remaining stammers will be much less tense than they were. This is the time to give yourself a pat on the back and to realize that the difficult part of therapy has been mastered.

The second part of therapy, you will remember, is to make the easy-stammers closer and closer to normal speech. We do this by gradually cutting down the length of the easy-stammers. Never try to decrease the length of a semi-easy-stammer which still has some tension in it. If your perfect easy-stammers last, say, about one and a half seconds, now begin to make them rather shorter – about one second; do not try to make them so short that they are not detectable. What I say can only be a guide, as every individual is different from every other individual, but the purpose is gradually to make the easy-stammers shorter on those controlled words which are now completely free of tension. If, after some weeks of practice, you find that you are successful in making the easy-stammers shorter, then do the same again, bringing them down to, say, half a second. But two words of warning: firstly, whenever tension appears in a word always *lengthen* the first syllable of that word and, secondly, never try to control a word without any lengthening at all.

As your control improves in the easier speaking situations, you will find that you are better able to exercise control in any remaining difficult situations, but, whatever the situation, you must work first at easy-stammering without tension before you begin to cut down on the lengthening. If you are finally able to cut down your easy-stammers to, say, half a second, I would not attempt to cut down any more. Half a second of lengthening is barely perceptible and, if you achieve something like that, you should practise it conscientiously for months before trying to decrease the lengthening still further. You may then find, in some situations anyway, that your control is so excellent that your listeners are quite unaware of the fact that you are controlling would-be-stammers because what they hear is normal speech.

13

Some Individual Problems

How use doth breed a habit in a man.

William Shakespeare

It would be wonderful indeed if the theory of easy-stammering always worked out 100 per cent in practice. Just occasionally it does, but it is very infrequently that people control so well, all the time, that no sign of stammer is ever heard again.

People, being people, tend to make two mistakes against all advice and evidence. Firstly, if they are naturally quick speakers, they often go on speaking too quickly, especially when they are excited. It is plainly impossible to easy-stammer if speech is rapid. Secondly, once people have learned to easy-stammer, they want and they try to cut out immediately any lengthening of the easy-stammer, but in so doing the tension returns. However, even if you make neither of these mistakes, you may find that some sounds, or groups of sounds, present real problems.

Some people, no matter how well they have learned the theory, sometimes have difficulty in getting a word started. I do not find this at all surprising because I believe that the original cause of the stammer is not eradicated by treatment. The 'core' of stammering appears to remain even when the bulk of the stammer has disappeared and the remainder is well controlled. Thus it is that the theory cannot always be applied completely successfully in practice. However, if you are unable to initiate speech because of blocking at the level of the larynx, it is very helpful to breathe in as this breaks the block and gives you a second chance; it is, of course, necessary to use the easy-stammer on your second attempt to initiate speech or you may block again. Taking a *deep* breath may upset the breathing pattern; it is best to breathe in naturally.

Any remaining problem sounds, on which you have so far been unable to easy-stammer successfully, will now be explained in more detail, and intensive practice in the correct manner virtually always makes it possible to easy-stammer on any sound. We will take these sounds in groups so that I can tell you how to cope with them.

The nasal sounds, 'm' and 'n'.

'M' often gives a great deal of trouble. This is because people push with their lips, creating tension. The lips should act only as a closed door; there must be no pressure between them. You *must* allow 'm' to come through your nose – that is its only possible exit! Let it come out in the form of a little hum (spoken, not sung) and hang on to it just for a second or two. If you are stuck on 'mine', for example, make a definite 'm' before you begin on the 'ine'. You cannot make the 'm' in a split second; you have got to give it time to come through your nose and if you do this properly you will feel slight vibrations in your nose. Once you have the right idea, you must start practising, to teach yourself how to do it. Take a list of words beginning with 'm'; make the 'm' long and then glide onto the sounds which follow, and remember to easy-stammer on the whole of the first syllable, not just the 'm'. Practise like this: 'm..o..ther', 'm..e..lody', 'm..a..ke', 'm..u..sic', and so on.

A similar approach should be used with 'n', except that the tip of the tongue is against the teeth ridge; make sure there is no pressure and that you allow 'n' to come through your nose. Say a long 'n' a few times, then practise it in words, e.g. 'n..o..se', 'n..e..ver', 'n..igh..tingale', 'n..a..tural'.

The vowel sounds

Remember that for all vowel sounds there is a freeway of air coming up from the lungs and through your mouth; there is no obstruction anywhere. If you cannot get started on some words beginning with vowels it is probably because there is tension at the level of the larynx. It is usually possible to master this problem by practising saying the vowel sounds with a continuant consonant in front of them, and later dropping the consonant; nonsense words in the early stages are easier to say than real words.

First, make a list of all the vowel sounds which give you trouble. I am going to suppose that 'ah' is one of the problem vowels, and I am choosing to put 'm' in front of it. You should practise, one at a time, in the way I shall describe, each vowel sound which is on your list:

1. Long 'm..' gliding on to long 'ah..' = 'm..ah..'; say this at least a dozen times, slowly and gently.
2. Next, add another lengthened 'ah' like this, 'm..ah..ah..', and say that several times also.
3. Next, with the lengthened 'ah', say some nonsense words such as 'ah..l..', 'ah..p', 'ah..sh..', 'ah..th..'.
4. Then, still with the easy-stammer, say some real words, e.g. 'ah..ch..' (arch), 'ah..m..y' (army), 'ah..n..ty' (aunty), and so on.

When you can do these successfully, you should do some reading practice; pick out all the words which begin with any vowels which were on your list, and deliberately easy-stammer on each one. You should do several hours of reading before attempting to use easy-stammering on your vowels in speech.

The letter 'h'

This sound does not often appear to cause trouble, but when it does it frequently causes quite severe stammering. I am reluctant to call it a sound because it is really just a puff of air. If you take in a deep breath and then let it out in a series of little voiceless sighs you will have produced a lot of little 'h' sounds. Once my patients discover that this sound is just a puff of air it is usually quite a short step for them to learn how to glide onto a vowel after it, so long as the vowel is lengthened in the usual way, e.g. 'h..ah..', 'h..ay..', 'h..ee..', 'h..oo..'. Practice on these should be followed by practice on real words, e.g. 'h..a..ppy', 'h..o..liday', 'h..ou..se', 'h..o..spital'. Later, the sound should be practised in reading in the usual way and, later still, it should be gently incorporated into speech.

The plosives

It seems to me that these six sounds, 'p', 'b', 't', 'd', 'k', 'g', or some of them, are stammered on more than any other group and are more difficult to control. I believe this is because of the complete blockage somewhere in the organs of speech which is required for their articulation; it seems that the tension tends to build up more when there is no freeway of air. Most people cope with plosives very well, using the method which I have described in the previous chapter, but I was aware for many years that not everybody could control their stammer adequately on the plosive sounds with the normal easy-stammer method. Quite recently I thought of a new way of coping with plosives, which I refer to as the 'new-look plosive', and, although most of my patients prefer the old method, at least two of them called the new look 'a break-through'.

You will recall that for the plosives the air stream is completely sealed off at some point; our problem is that when this happens there is a tendency for tension to build up in the organs of speech which are employed in the process of sealing off. Let us first take 'p' and 'b'; the two lips are together and air pressure is building up behind them, in order to produce the appropriate sound when the lips are exploded apart. With the 'new look' you do not let the air pressure build up. You put your lips together in the usual way but only actually pronounce the remainder of the word (with the usual lengthening of the first syllable, of course). So, if you are going to say 'bike', you just put your lips together and say 'ike'. Of course, it is possible for you deliberately to say just the 'ike', but if you practise correctly you will find that as you part your two lips there is a tiny 'b' sound as you glide on to the 'i..ke'. Once you can manage this you should do the same thing with a word beginning with 'p', e.g. 'pebble'. Put your lips together and, as you part them, you should glide on to a lengthened 'e..bble'. Next, take a list of words beginning with 'p' and 'b' and practise them in the manner I have described.

Next you should practise the new-look plosive on the sounds 't' and 'd'. Try the two words 'take' and 'dear'. Put your tongue in the correct position for 't' and, with no pressure, glide on to 'a..ke'. Keep on doing it until 't' can just be heard. Then do the same with 'd' gliding on to 'ea..r'. Follow this by practising on a list of words beginning with 't' and 'd', and be sure to remember to lengthen the vowel which follows.

The sounds 'k' and 'g' are treated in the same manner except that the speech organs are in a different position. Put your tongue in the right position for 'k' and then say 'i..ng' (king); if only the 'i..ng' can be heard, keep working at it until a tiny 'k' glides on to the rest of the word. Then do the same for 'g': have your tongue ready for 'g' and then follow it by saying 'a..le' (gale). If you can hear only the 'a..le', try again and again until the gentle 'g' glides on to the 'a..le'. Then practise this from word lists.

It will be appreciated that in the early stages of using the new-look plosive it is necessary to slow down the word you are trying to control, because it takes a lot of concentration and also cannot be done successfully if hurried. I therefore advise you, once you are able to cope with the plosives in this way, to practise a great deal on your own and with close friends before you begin trying to use it in public; once you have had plenty of practice you will find that you can speed up considerably.

If the plosive sound should be immediately followed by another consonant, it sounds most natural if you give that consonant just a little lengthening, and keep the greatest lengthening on the vowel sound, e.g. 'bread' = lips in 'b' position followed by 'r.ea..d'; 'driving = tongue in 'd' position followed by 'r.i..ving'; 'glove' = tongue in 'g' position followed by 'l.o..ve'.

The sounds 'ch' (chair) and 'j' (jar)

These sounds, if broken down phonetically, are actually two sounds which follow each other in such rapid succession that they are heard as one sound. Both of them are made up of a plosive followed by a continuant. In the case of 'ch' it is a 't' followed by 'sh'; 'j' is made up of 'd' followed by the sound 's' in 'measure'.

My purpose in explaining this in detail is to help you understand that you may have to treat these sounds as plosives, instead of continuants, when you easy-stammer on them. Usually people can treat them as continuants but occasionally these two sounds continue to cause a lot of tension. When this happens you should regard them as plosive sounds and deal with them in the manner described in the previous chapter.

The semi-vowels, 'w' and 'y'

If these sounds continue to give you trouble, despite the fact that you have attempted conscientiously to easy-stammer on them, it is almost certain that you are trying to say them too quickly. If you *are* trying to say them too quickly you should get into the habit of regarding 'w' as 'oo' and 'y' as 'ee'. First, take a list of nonsense words and (on your own, until you get some success) make the 'oo' and 'ee' excessively long, e.g. 'oo——ah', 'oo——ay', 'oo——ee', 'oo——o'; 'ee——ah', 'ee——ay', 'ee——o', 'ee——oo'.

After a considerable amount of practice you should do the same thing with real words. Later, go over everything you have already done but make the 'oo' and 'ee' a little shorter. Later still, when you try to use these sounds in your conversation, watch yourself carefully so that you can see when they are going to occur in your speech, and try to easy-stammer on them before the tension begins, thinking of the two sounds as 'oo' and 'ee'.

The sounds 'f', 'v', 'th', 's', 'z', 'sh'

These continuant consonants are called 'fricatives' because in their production there is a narrowing of the mouth passage and, as the air is forced through it, there is audible friction.

Sometimes people stammer so severely on some of these

sounds (especially 's' and 'f') that they run out of breath before getting off them, and, even after another or several more breaths, the sound continues to be prolonged or repeated before the rest of the word eventually comes out. I shall take 's' as my example in helping you to deal with your problem, although what I say applies to all the sounds in this group. I choose 's' because I have so often heard people struggling with it for long periods and then learning, in just a few minutes, how to get off the 's' and on to the remainder of the word.

The first thing to be aware of is that once you have started saying 's' you have already said all that is required. Whether, when you stammer on it, you prolong the sound (i.e. sssssssssssss) or whether you continue to repeat the sound (s-s-s-s-s-s-s-s-s-s-s-s), in either case there is no need to say more than the first 's'. Your problem is to get off the 's' instead of continuing with it, so first practise saying it just one 's' and then stopping everything. You don't *have* to go on and on saying 's' so long as you get used to the idea that you are capable of stopping it as soon as you start, and by that time you have already said a complete 's'.

Your next job is to follow a single 's' with a vowel, and this can usually be done so long as you concentrate on making the vowel long. To start with, forget about words (because you have trained yourself to know that 's' words are often impossible for you) and concentrate only on the individual sounds. Think of one 's' and the sound 'oa' and the sound 'p' and then say them slowly one after the other, 's..oa..p'; do the same with 's..i..t'; then with 's..igh..t'. The most important thing to concentrate on is the lengthening of the vowel sound which follows the 's'. Then make the usual list of words and practise those in the same way, always gently and slowly. When you start to use your easy-stammer 's' in conversation, begin by deliberately doing it on some of the words which begin with 's'; that is, fake it. This will help you to get used to doing it; we use the sound 's' so much in our speech that it is difficult to cope with every 's' but this is made easier if you have already had some success with it through faking it.

The sounds 'l' and 'r'

These are the only two remaining sounds which we have not covered in dealing with individual problems. Normally they can be controlled in the usual way of easy-stammering. If they do, however, present a particular problem they should be managed in the same way as the previous group of sounds, that is, by saying one single 'l' or one single 'r' followed by a lengthened vowel sound. You must concentrate on lengthening the vowel, which helps you to get off the 'l' or the 'r'.

Excessive speed of speech

This is a frequent problem, which we have already discussed. Most people can slow down their speech if they really set their minds to it, but I believe that if you are naturally a fast talker you always have a tendency to speak too fast, which means that you have to be vigilant. If you can get into the habit of *beginning* any conversation with slowed down speech, you will find that it is easier to keep to that rate for the whole conversation; if you start a conversation with rapid speech, it is harder to slow down for that particular conversation. If too rapid speech presents a constant problem, it is often very helpful to practise slow reading, where you can only see one word at a time. To do this, you should cut a corner out of a post-card and place it on the reading material so that you can only see one word; you must finish saying that word before moving the card along so that you can see the second word, then finish saying the second word before moving the card along so that you can see the third word, and so on. This makes reading extremely slow and is also very boring to do. If you are serious about it, you will make yourself do this for one hour daily and this should remind you to talk more slowly. If it does not remind you, you should increase the slow-reading time by half an hour. If you still do not succeed, you should go on increasing the slow-reading time; in the end it gets so time-consuming and so monotonous that it is easier to remember to talk more slowly than it is to spend all those hours on 'corner-out-of-card' reading.

Sometimes people who speak quickly manage to slow down their speech very well in order to acquire the easy-stammer, and achieve almost perfect fluency in many situations. With the increased fluency, however, their speech speeds up again and when this happens the tension returns, so once you have achieved a reasonable rate of speaking it is necessary to maintain that rate and not return to the original too-fast speech.

Reminders

Sometimes, although you are quite capable of easy-stammering, you simply forget to do it. You finish a conversation and then realize that you have stammered and have quite forgotten about the easy-stammer. This should act as a reminder to easy-stammer in your next conversation, but there are other things you can use to remind you. You can make up your own reminders which should be related to the things which you do during your usual day; when you see your reminder to easy-stammer, don't just give it a passing glance but spend a few seconds concentrating on it. You should put a notice somewhere which you will see first thing in the morning, e.g. on your shaving mirror or beside your clock, saying, 'Remember to easy-stammer today.' If you smoke filter-tip cigarettes, put them upside-down in the packet so that every time you take one out it reminds you. If you drive, tie a piece of string on the steering wheel; if you use the telephone frequently, put a piece of sticky-tape on it; if you use a brief-case, put a strip of coloured sellotape inside the lid so that you are reminded each time you open it; if you use pens or pencils often, put different coloured rubber bands round each one. If you do these things, you will find they are a great aid to remembering, so long as you concentrate on them when you see them. After a while the reminders will probably wear thin, and when this happens you need to change them.

If the use of reminders is not sufficient to help you remember to easy-stammer as much as you should, then every night you need to write a list of the situations in which you remembered to easy-stammer and the situations in which you did not. This daily assessment of your successes and failures should make you more aware, in future, of the situations in which you forgot to easy-stammer.

14

Easy-Stammering for Children

*Children and watches must not be constantly wound up –
you must let them run.*

Jean Paul

We have already discussed those little children who stammer before school age, when the environment can be controlled. In this chapter I want to talk about children, of all other ages, who are aware that they have a speech problem and want to do something about it.

It is impossible to say what precisely should be done for any particular age-group because children vary so much in degree of awareness of stammer, in desire to overcome it, in understanding of what to do about it, and in ability to do it. Generally speaking, I use easy-stammering for all age-groups; it is my explanation of it that varies, according to the age and understanding of any particular child. Usually (but by no means always) a child's stammer is less complicated than that of an adult, which enables me to keep my explanations of therapy as simple as possible. What I say about children must, therefore, be taken as general and not specific.

Age twelve or over

At this age most children are quite capable of understanding the difference between a continuant and a plosive, and of learning how to apply the easy-stammer to these two different groups of sounds (as explained in Chapter 12, and, if necessary, Chapter 13). Therapy is much the same for children in this age-group as for adults, and they learn, by experience in both reading and speaking, that it is possible to control the stammer instead of being controlled by it. As the child is usually brought by his mother, I tell her all about easy-stammering too, so that she knows exactly what he is trying to do. I expect the child to do daily reading practice, first for faking and later for converting, and then gradually to incorporate easy-stammering into speaking situations. We make the usual list of situations, from the easiest to those which are most difficult for him, and work through these one after the other, just as for the adults. Usually children prefer to use the easy-stammer at home and with their friends at first, then with the other children at school and later with their most-liked teachers, before using it with their least-liked teachers.

When a child is learning to easy-stammer at home, I find it is extremely helpful for him and his mother to sit down together every day and have a conversation in which he concentrates on using the easy-stammer. His mother must fully understand that it is much easier to use in reading than in speech, and that it is not always possible to control the stammer despite the will to do so. This practice must be carried out at a suitable time of the day, when they are alone and unhurried. Later, when the child is able to easy-stammer at home, but forgets to do so, his mother may remind him by saying an agreed word such as 'oy' or 'steady', but she should not become emotionally involved when he forgets.

Instead of assessing stammer improvement in terms of frequency, duration, and severity, as for adults, I usually talk about the two piles of 'I can' and 'I can't'. When he first came to the clinic he could not control any of the stammers so the pile of 'I can' did not exist. Now, every single time he controls a stammer, without any tension at all, the 'I can' pile grows a little bit bigger and the 'I can't' pile grows a little bit smaller. When he draws the two piles he can judge for himself what the difference is; then a few months later he can draw them again to see if there is further improvement, remembering to take into account all the different situations in which he speaks.

Children aged from approximately six to eleven years

The whole purpose of learning to easy-stammer in the clinic is that the child shall eventually be able to use easy-stammering in all situations; the more he talks without tension, the more the stammer decreases. With small children, however, I do not work on trying to use the easy-stammer in one situation after another; rather I try to give them the knowledge, through experience, that it is possible to talk without tension.

While the therapy for even small children is basically the same as that for adults, I explain things rather differently. I do not use the term 'easy-stammering' at all, but call it 'elastic words'. Neither do I mention syllables or distinguish between different groups of sounds. I only call his stammer a stammer if that is what he calls it; if he says, 'The words get stuck', I refer to it as 'when the words get stuck'; if he says, 'The words take a long time', I refer to it as 'when the words take a long time'. For faking elastic words in reading or in speech, I use the phrase 'doing elastic words on purpose', and for converting true stammers to easy ones I use the phrase 'changing the hard words into elastic ones'.

I teach easy-stammering by saying that if one stretches out the first part of the word, like a piece of elastic, it is nearly always possible to get the word out easily. We then start practising to prove it. I ask him to tell me some of the words that are difficult and he might say 'mmmmmmummy' and 'ssssssschool', each with a real stammer. Then I tell him that we will try saying them the elastic way; I say 'm..u..mmy' and he repeats it, almost always without tension and very often with a surprised grin. Then I say 's..choo..l' the elastic way, and so does he. We do several words like this until he has the idea; when he cannot remember any more difficult words, we practise on any single words. Once this can be done, we begin reading for practice. If he is able to read, he stretches out the first part of the first word of each line; if he is too young to read, he copies me doing it. It helps in the early stages to underline the first words with coloured ink. Just as for the adults, we concentrate to start with only on the first word of each line, to make the word elastic; true stammers on other words are ignored for the time being. Then a few weeks later, we stop and change any true stammers in reading to elastic words; later still, we practise on the first word of each line plus any true stammers along the rest of the line.

I explain the therapy to the mother in some detail and, in the early stages of treatment, she spends some of the time with us, so that she can hear her child using elastic words and thus understand how it gets rid of the tension. Throughout treatment I always have a few minutes with her to find out what progress or problems she has to report, and also to tell her what we have been working on during our session. If both mother and child are willing to do a few minutes' daily homework, I ask them to practise elastic reading and/or have a talk together, both using elastic words some of the time. I discourage correction of true stammers in general conversation except for those children who are very willing to be reminded to use elastic words when they are 'stuck'. Some children correct themselves when true stammers occur, but this is the exception rather than the rule in the early stages of treatment.

Each week I ask the child and his mother to make a list of the words which have been really difficult for him to say. I give him a little book for this purpose which he can also use for drawing or anything else he likes, to make it a 'fun' book. When he returns with his list of hard words, we play a game in which I say each word (one at a time) the hard way and he repeats them the elastic way, then he says them the hard way and I repeat them the elastic way. Children really enjoy doing this.

Sometimes I find it helpful to play any game in which both the child and I deliberately say some of the words the hard way; when this happens the other person has to immediately repeat that word the elastic way. This helps the child to become aware of true stammers because it is essential to really concentrate on speech in order to play the game, and with the added concentration he is often able to control true stammers.

After the first few weeks of therapy, I try to incorporate five things in any one session:

1. Any conversation about his interests, with no interruption on my part, and no reaction to any stammers.
2. Playing the elastic game with his word list.
3. Reading for elastic word practice.
4. Conversation or games for elastic word practice, either 'doing elastic words on purpose' or changing real stammers to easy ones, in which I am allowed to interrupt.
5. Having a talk with the child's mother about what we have done, and how she can help until he comes again.

Different approaches are necessary for different children, however. One child might talk so much that it is necessary to curtail the chat somewhat in order to get in some practice; another may talk so little that one has to improvise by playing games in which we both use elastic words.

For a child who has to read aloud at school, and who stammers when he is doing it, a lot can be done. If he practises deliberately using elastic words on the first two or three words of any reading passage, he is usually off to a good start and more able to continue without stammer; if much stammering occurs later in the reading, he needs a lot of practice in the clinic, and at home, starting off the first two or three words of each *sentence* with elastic words. Then, when he has more confidence in his ability to control when reading, he should attempt to put it into practice at school. Sometimes it may be necessary to ask his teacher to excuse him from reading but this still makes him 'different', and it is much better for him to continue his reading if he is able, in this way, to control his stammer.

Before starting on elastic word therapy for children, one might wonder to what extent the syllable should be 'stretched'. The fact is that the children who manage to use this method find their own level. They usually make it quite long (perhaps a second or more) in reading practice but tend to make it rather briefer in speech. It should be long enough to be free of tension but not so long as to be embarrassing for the child. As with all age groups, it gets briefer with practice.

If you are the parent of a child who has a stammer and intend to help him to replace it by this method, I would strongly advise you also to consult a speech therapist. When you are treating a child for his stammer you have to make him a little bit conscious of it, but this should be carried only to the extent that he is interested in doing something about it. If you go too far or push too hard you are liable to make him over-aware of his stammer, which could increase it and also decrease his confidence. A parent and a speech therapist together should be able to work out how much direct work can be done on the stammer for any individual child.

15

Some Results of Easy-Stammering

The winds and waves are always on the side of the ablest navigators.

Edward Gibbon

Ever since I began to teach easy-stammering I have known that it brings good results to the patients who really work at achieving it, but I did not try to measure what degrees of success were achieved. In 1972 I decided to get in touch with as many as possible of the adult patients who had attended the clinic for therapy during the ten years from 1960 to 1969, inclusive;* the gap of anything between two and twelve years since they had learned easy-stammering gave plenty of opportunity for relapse, if any had in fact occurred.

During those ten years (when I was still working just one weekly session for adults) eighty-seven patients with stammers were referred to me and all were offered easy-stammering therapy. Of these eighty-seven, twenty-four people attended on fewer than ten occasions and were therefore regarded as not serious in their aim; thirteen left the district or went abroad; thirteen more asked for a different type of therapy. This left thirty-seven people who attended regularly, or at least on more than ten occasions, for easy-stammering therapy; I wrote to all of them and received replies from twenty-six but was unable to contact the remaining eleven. In summary:

Number of patients referred for treatment, 1960–69	87
Number who attended for fewer than ten sessions	24
Number who left the district	13

*A. Irwin, 'The Treatment and Results of "Easy-Stammering"', *British Journal of Disorders of Communication*, 7, 2, pp. 151–6, 1972.

Some Results of Easy-Stammering · 107

Number who asked for a different therapy	13

Therefore:

Number who attended regularly for easy-stammering therapy	37
Replies received to my letters of inquiry	26
Of the 26 people who replied, number subsequently interviewed	18

To the twenty-six who replied, I sent questionnaires which read as follows:

Improvement of a stammer can be measured in FOUR ways:
1. *Frequency* of stammer, i.e. how often the stammers occur.
2. *Duration* of stammer, i.e. the actual length of time that the stammers take.
3. *Severity* of stammer, i.e. how severe the stammers are.
4. *Attitude* towards stammering, i.e. less worry about it, more confidence when speaking.

In the FOUR boxes below, kindly enter the number which indicates the change in your stammer since you started 'easy-stammering':

1. No change.
2. *Duration* of stammer, i.e. the actual length of time that the
3. Good improvement.
4. Very good improvement.
5. Excellent improvement (i.e. very little stammer now).
6. Complete improvement (i.e. no stammer now).

FREQUENCY 1–6	DURATION 1–6	SEVERITY 1–6	ATTITUDE 1–6

Also on the questionnaire was a space for 'remarks', and a note was sent inviting each patient to visit me, if he was willing and it was possible, so that I could judge for myself whether his assessment of the improvement in his stammer corresponded to my own assessment of his improvement. Of these twenty-six people, I was able to interview eighteen; the majority of the eight whom I was unable to see had left the district.

I felt satisfied after seeing these eighteen people, talking with them at some length, and listening to what they said about their speech outside the clinical situation that, apart from one man (no. 18 on the chart on pages 110–11) who, I thought, rather overestimated his improvement, and two others (nos. 12 and 26) who, I thought, underestimated their improvement, each of them had made a valid assessment of his improvement as regards the frequency, duration, and severity of his stammer, and also as regards his attitude towards it. The chart shows the results obtained.

The chart is self-explanatory and needs only a little comment. The twenty-six individual results are shown, and it will be seen that the average assessment is 'very good improvement' as regards the frequency and the duration of the stammer, and between 'very good improvement' and 'excellent improvement' as regards the severity of the stammer and the attitude towards stammering.

The average number of attendances at the clinic was thirty-five. The average number of years of attendance is not meaningful because, in some cases, students attended a few times and then left Newcastle for vacations, so that therapy was intermittent, and in other cases, some patients attended a few times and then failed to attend, only to turn up months later to 'try again'. In most cases patients attended weekly to begin with, alternately individually for half an hour and in a group for one hour. When they felt confident enough, they just attended the group once fortnightly. They were discharged either because both they and I felt that their stammer was now socially acceptable, and that they would not benefit from further therapy (twenty), or because they were leaving the district (six).

It is of interest that the three patients (nos. 1, 8, and 16), all professional people, who averaged seventy-seven visits each, did not make the effort required to use easy-stammering; neither do they rank high in stammer improvement. Elimination of these three patients would bring down the number of attendances, by the remaining twenty-three patients, to an average of thirty visits each.

No. 1 wrote on her questionnaire, 'This is an easily learned technique which only needs practice to perfect. My failing is that I have not practised sufficiently, so that when I get into difficulties I am unable to use it.'

No. 8 wrote, 'I still often find myself in the situation of being "caught out", i.e. stammering before I realize it, and it is then more difficult to apply the easy-stammer.'

No. 16 (after ninety-six visits) said, 'I could not remember, in precise terms, exactly what easy-stammering is. Having had it explained to me again, I can say that I use it in some, but not most, situations.'

Quotes from a few other patients show that they had achieved a far greater success:

No. 12: 'Nine times out of ten I don't stammer at all; it is not a big problem in my life any more. I gave a twenty-minute speech in front of thirty people at college, and didn't stammer at all. I still choose my words a bit, and find reading to people more difficult than talking.'

No. 9: 'I do not have to easy-stammer when talking to friends and relatives as I almost always speak very well in these situations. I think my best improvement has been in the attitude – I am no longer terrified to go into shops, etc.'

No. 11: 'I have gone on improving over the years since I left. If you think before you speak, it's quite easy, so long as you use the easy-stammer. Most of the time the stammer is seldom and brief. I never worry now and I never get blocks.'

No. 10: 'The easy-stammer is not needed. I feel that I no longer stammer. I can talk to fifty patients a day, and probably don't hesitate more than once. It has certainly changed my life.'

The reader of this attempt to measure improvement of stammering will study the chart and read what people say about themselves, but the figures will remain figures rather than bring to life the people who worked on their speech and who, as they did so, grew in confidence and in fluency. Perhaps I may conclude this chapter by writing out part of a conversation taken from a tape recording of two students who were making their

Survey of patients taught easy-stammering 1960–69*

Patients	Frequency (1–6)†	Duration (1–6)†	Severity (1–6)†	Attitude (1–6)†
1	3	3	3	4
2	5	5	5	5
3	5	5	5	5
4	4	5	4	5
5	3	2	5	3
6	4	5	5	4
7	5	5	5	6
8	2	3	2	3
9	4	5	6	5
10	6	6	6	6
11	5	5	5	5
12	4	2	3	3
13	1	2	3	3
14	5	5	6	5
15	4	4	5	6
16	3	2	3	4
17	5	5	5	5
18	5	5	5	6
19	5	5	5	5
20	5	5	5	6
21	3	2	3	5
22	3	5	5	4
23	3	4	4	5
24	3	3	3	4
25	3	3	3	4
26	3	2	3	2
Average:	3.9	4	4.3	4.5

*From A. Irwin, 'The Treatment and Results of "Easy-Stammering"', op. cit.

†Numbers represent graded performance as follows:
1. No change.
2. Slight improvement.
3. Good improvement.
4. Very good improvement.
5. Excellent improvement (i.e. very little stammer now).
6. Complete improvement (i.e. no stammer now).

Some Results of Easy-Stammering · 111

Sex	Total Attendances (Number)	(Years)	Present Age (Years)	Seen or Not Seen
F	81	4	35	Seen
M	41	2	35	Seen
M	31	2	35	Seen
M	17	2	31	Seen
M	24	2	34	Not seen
M	38	2	26	Not Seen
M	17	2	25	Seen
M	55	4	44	Not seen
M	20	1	17	Not seen
M	50	3	24	Seen
M	20	2	29	Seen
M	33	1	26	Seen
M	11	1	21	Seen
M	25	2	25	Not Seen
M	38	2	21	Seen
M	96	4	38	Seen
M	50	3	37	Seen
M	47	3	52	Seen
M	10	1	28	Seen
M	25	1	23	Seen
M	21	1	37	Not seen
M	26	2	23	Not Seen
M	11	1	22	Seen
M	41	2	23	Seen
M	50	3	38	Not seen
M	37	2	37	Seen
	35			

last visit to the clinic, before leaving Newcastle for jobs elsewhere.

Me (to Mr B): 'Tell me just one thing – do you not stammer at all now? I haven't heard you stammer yet.'

Mr B: 'I've stammered, I think I've counted about six times' (i.e. perfect control).

Me: 'Since you've been in here?'

Mr B: 'Since, yes.'

Me: 'Have you? How many' (to Miss A.) 'stammers have *you* noticed – any?'

Miss A: 'Well, I don't think I've noticed any at all, to tell you the truth; I'm not just saying that but it's marvellous.'

Mr B: 'Well the same goes for you – I haven't heard any at all; I don't know what *you* think.'

Miss A: 'Well I think my speech has improved a hell of a lot since I've been coming to the R.V.I.'*

Me: 'I think it will last now because you've had so many periods away – dropping in, and coming back after long vacations – and it's been maintained for quite a while now, hasn't it?'

Miss A: 'Oh yes it has, yes. You know I still get setbacks, but overall, it's much better than it was because it's a constructive method. I mean, you can *do* something about it. I think the thing about easy-stammering is that it's constructive. All the methods I've been taught in the past – I mean – they've been a help and they've restored my confidence but they've not been practical enough; they've not told me what to do with the plosives and what to do with the so-and-so's, and I think this is what I really needed, something more practical, and it's been marvellous.'

*Royal Victoria Infirmary.

Section Three

16

Speak for Yourself

'Tis not in mortals to command success,
But we'll do more . . . ; we'll deserve it.

Joseph Addison

I know that the therapy of easy-stammering is not the complete answer, nor anywhere near the complete answer, to the problem of stammering. With the exception of children, when my patients stop attending for treatment, either by choice or by mutual agreement, their stammers have never been totally eliminated. What stammer remains is a very much smaller problem, but it may still be considered to be a problem.

Yet this simple and direct approach does bring very considerable alleviation and, being so simple and straightforward, it brings the possibility of stammer control within the grasp of anybody who is willing and able to work on his speech.

In this chapter, where my patients 'speak for themselves', it should be remembered that I do not select the people who would be most likely to benefit from therapy, and none of my patients have been excluded except for the few who repeatedly say that, for various reasons, they mostly fail to work on their speech. I must also point out that I am not measuring stammer improvement in the clinical situation, where speech is frequently at its best; nor am I speaking for other people.

Instead, I have asked all of my current patients who work fairly or very conscientiously on trying to control their stammers to write an account of what easy-stammering means to them and how much it has helped them so far. To complete the picture, I have also asked a few patients who have been recently discharged to do the same.

At the time of writing, I have sixteen adults and eleven young people of sixteen years or under coming for therapy. Some attend regularly; others periodically. Some come to the group; others come individually. Of the sixteen adults, three 'mostly fail to work on their speech', and are therefore not included in this report. Of the eleven young people, three 'mostly fail'. The other eight (or their mothers) have been asked to speak for themselves about their progress. In so doing, some patients mention the benefits of 'speaking slowly'. They do not, in fact, speak slowly and it would have been more accurate to have said 'speaking more slowly' or 'speaking less rapidly'.

This is what they say.

Adults

1. MR A.B. (AGE: EIGHTEEN)
When I first started speech therapy at the R.V.I. over three months ago my speech was never stammer-free, but the stammer varied in different situations, and some sounds were harder than others. Now using the easy-stammer technique, in most situations, I am achieving a much easier flow of words.

Before easy-stammering I was not very keen to speak on the telephone, but I am now just beginning to employ this technique on the telephone, and I now do not mind that situation in the least.

As a child I had several years of speech therapy with only limited success.

2. MR B.C. (AGE: TWENTY-EIGHT)
Since my first attendance at speech therapy nine weeks ago, I have found that easy-stammering has helped me to get over previously difficult situations, which I tended to avoid, or at least tried to avoid. This has been achieved, I believe, by an increase in confidence given by the knowledge that at least I now know what to do if I feel that I am going to stammer.

A list of difficult speaking situations was compiled. These were ten in number and were listed in order of difficulty, starting with the easiest. To date I am using easy-stammering in four of these situations, which included ordering a beer, which is called 'Special', at my local. This was difficult due to my stammer being more pronounced when 's' is followed by a plosive. However, after having been taught the easy-stammer method, this particular situation became less difficult as my experience and confidence grew. This has proved the case with the other three situations in which I have worked. As experience in these situations increases, I find that I need not concentrate to the same degree as was at first required.

As my occupation is a Police Constable the easy-stammer has proved particularly helpful when interviewing persons in connection with my work, in particular saying words where 's' is followed by a plosive, either at the beginning or in the middle of words, for example, '*s*tatement' and 'in*s*pector'.

The most difficult part of the therapy to conquer, I have found and still find, is 'to speak more slowly and to concentrate'. But I find that if I speak slower it is easier to concentrate.

3. MR R.D. (AGE: FORTY-SIX)

I am forty-six and have been stammering for as long as I can remember. Three years prior to going for treatment it got a lot worse. I was finding it increasingly difficult to communicate with people outside of my immediate family circle. This caused me to dread simple things like going into shops and travelling on buses. I constantly feared experiencing a block in those situations, and when making conversation I tried to switch words to avoid stammering.

I went to see my doctor to see if he could do anything for me. He said that there was nothing he personally could do, but he would put me in touch with a speech therapist. On my first visit to the clinic it was explained to me that there was no magic cure, however the therapist could help me if I was prepared to help myself. The method to be used was easy-stammering within a group of people who had the same problem. At first I found it very difficult and progress was slow until I absorbed the technique and began to think to use it all the time. My first success was in the home with my family which was an easy situation. I began to find that I would rather easy-stammer than switch words. This led eventually to my using easy-stammering in the hard situations, i.e. in shops and buses.

Although it did not stop me from stammering completely, my speech was socially acceptable and I found talking to strangers much easier. This made a big difference to my life; things which I once dreaded I no longer have any fear of. It is two years since I started the clinic; after one year of weekly attendance my visits were tailed off on the therapist's advice. I only occasionally attend now as my speech remains socially acceptable.

4. MRS J.H. (AGE: TWENTY-NINE)

I started stammering at the age of three years old, but previous therapy while still at school did not help much. From the age of fourteen years until three years ago, I had no therapy at all for my stammer. I stammered in all situations but mostly when saying my own name and the names of my family. I avoided using the telephone as much as I could.

I had to slow down my speech quite a bit and this helped me to overcome some of my stammer. Lengthening the words by easy-stammering has helped me a great deal as it gives me more confidence when talking to people. It took me quite a while to remember to easy-stammer when talking, but once I got into the way of it, it is always in the back of my mind.

I found nasal sounds and plosives were the hardest to overcome, and I used to try and push the words out, until I found that, by saying the nasal sounds through my nose, they came out much easier and free of tension.

I used to avoid talking to people if at all possible, in the past, but now I even find it easier to make conversation to strangers. After five months of therapy about 50 per cent of my stammer had gone, as I had gained much more confidence than I previously had.

Phone calls have not got much better and I avoid phoning anywhere that I have to give my name, if at all possible. I can cope with incoming calls quite well. If I can pause for a few seconds before saying my name I can usually say it free of tension.

Within a year my speech was often stammer-free for a few days at a time. I have no difficulty in reading to my children, but I am not so good at reading out of a newspaper. I spent a few days in hospital and I had no bother saying my name.

I would say that about 80 to 85 per cent of my stammer has gone, and the remainder I can control if I remember to slow down and pause for a second or two before I speak. The situations which are usually stammer-free are when I have a general chat to relations and friends, when there appears to be no tension at hand.

Before attending therapy sessions I found life (conversation-wise) unbearable because of my inability to talk to people. The therapy sessions have given me untold confidence and in time perhaps I'll be 99 per cent cured of my stammer. I stopped regular attendance some time ago but still go to the group meetings occasionally.

5. MR G.J. (AGE: NINETEEN)

I first attended speech therapy nearly three years ago. Before I attended speech therapy my speech must have been bad; I say this because I was not aware of how bad it really was until I became more aware of my stammer. Speech therapy makes you more aware of your stammer, and thus you become more self-conscious of it and embarrassed talking to people, whereas before you just took it for granted.

During the first two years of therapy I was still at school and did not take it seriously; I only occasionally used easy-stammering in difficult situations, because of two reasons; one was I was afraid to use it because it sounded so artificial to me and thus, because I was afraid to use it, I tended to forget about it and just plod on with my speech.

After I left school I knew I was going to have to improve if I was going to stand any chance of getting a job. I re-attended speech therapy after a break of three months, with a new enthusiasm and attitude to controlling my stammer.

About three weeks after this I attended a number of interviews for jobs in which I spoke very well, speaking slowly and controlling my stammer. This gave me much needed confidence; now after six months' continual concentration in slowing down and easy-stammering my stammer has improved 80 per cent.

This new confidence has changed my whole outlook on life, speech-wise. Now I can stand up and speak, or ask questions in a crowded room at ease, whereas six months ago I would not have dared to do this.

Even though I have improved 80 per cent I still have a long way to go, because you can always feel the stammer there as you talk as if it was bursting to get out and show itself. Now I feel, though, I am controlling the stammer, and not as I felt before that the stammer was controlling me.

6. MR J.L. (AGE: EIGHTEEN)

I have had a stammer since I was six years of age. People laughed when I went into shops to buy things, but what I really hated was my friends laughing and this made me really mad. In fact some people, even today, still laugh, but these are just stupid people who do not know what it is like to have a stammer.

I have been out with a few girls but I have not been going steady because they think it is funny, and I am always serious about it. It is hard to describe in words what I mean to say.

I went to see my doctor and he decided that I should go to speech therapy. At first I was a bit nervous but I soon got over it, and it became like a habit going on a Tuesday; I was learning easy-stammer which was quite difficult but I soon got to know it – plosives, etc. This I thought was easy but then I didn't go for a few weeks and when I went back I was all to pieces, so I had to start again and it became harder for some reason; maybe I was not relaxed enough at this time. I got a part-time job in a pub which helped me quite a lot, and I made a lot of friends. I wouldn't have gone into the pub if it wasn't for easy-stammer, but since I got the job I have really worked hard to make my speech more fluent. Not so long ago I met some of my old school chums and they were amazed because they thought I had lost my stammer, so since learning about easy-stammer I have improved a lot.

7. MISS J.L. (AGE: NINETEEN)

It was certainly a weight off my mind when I was referred to someone who actually stuck to one method, and not several half-hearted attempts to eliminate my stammer; but I was also quite desperate and determined this time to do something about my speech. Whereas before I had always managed to get round or out of difficult situations, this time I had to try my hardest so as to be able to teach in primary schools.

I had never before been able to control my stammer, which for the most part was a series of tongue-thrusts and splutters, but with practice I learnt to easy-stammer in various situations. It was hard at first, especially with my fellow students, most of whom had little patience with the real stammer or the easy-stammer. But gradually I began talking more and stopped substituting easier-to-say words. The tongue thrust occurs very rarely now but there are still situations where, despite my attempts at easy-stammering, the tension is still there. The problems usually occur when the person I'm talking to is embarrassed, is impatient, finishes words or sentences off for me, or mocks me. But generally I can be confident that in most situations I can manage.

However, it must be remembered this is not a magic cure, but a method which brings results only with hard work and practice.

8. MR W.MC C. (AGE: THIRTY-NINE)

I began speech therapy ten months ago and since starting the class my family and friends have noticed a big change in my speech, about 80 per cent. When I talk slow and use easy-stammering, which helps me quite a lot, I can now speak to strangers. Talking slowly has almost got rid of the very bad habit I had of saying 'you know' every time I got stuck.

I haven't noticed any real blocks in my speech for the last few months; I used to close my eyes quite a lot when I couldn't get my words out, but I very rarely do this now.

I find I can talk much easier in the clinic now as I have gained quite a lot of confidence. At one time I would never go into a shop and ask for cigarettes; I would rather get them from a machine or get one of my friends to get them for me. I wouldn't go into a strange bar as I could never seem to ask for what I wanted and this used to embarrass me terribly. Whenever I had to go on a bus I always made sure I had the right change so that I needn't ask for my ticket, or if my wife was with me she would ask for the fares; now I am able to do this myself.

My workmates have noticed a great improvement in my speech; I can join in their conversations quite freely now – at one time I would just sit and listen, now I have my say. The only time I have noticed myself stammer is if I get excited.

Easy-stammering is the best thing that could have happened for me as it has given me all the confidence which I could never find on my own.

My brother-in-law came home from Scotland and I hadn't seen him for about six months; he asked me where my stammer had gone, to which I replied, 'the R.V.I. Speech Therapy'. Many thanks for the therapy which has helped me, and many others like myself, gain the confidence in themselves which they could never find before attending the class.

9. MR S.Q. (AGE: EIGHTEEN)

I cannot say much as I have been receiving treatment for only five weeks, but already there is an enormous improvement.

Before I started the treatment my stammer was really bad. I seemed to be making a squeaking noise in my throat when I was talking. I later found out that as I was finding it difficult to stammer on an out-breath, as anybody else would, I was trying to overcome this by stammering on an in-breath, which is virtually impossible, thus this squeaking noise was being produced.

On my first appointment I was introduced to 'easy-stammer', and told briefly what it was all about. I was also told my main troubles, and how we would work on these later on.

After only five weeks I am finding it easier to talk and the squeaking noise has almost gone.

10. MR P.R. (AGE: THIRTY-FOUR)

My earliest recollection of stammering is at the age of six; the one fact that I can associate it with this period of my life is an accident, in which I gashed my right knee, requiring fifteen stitches and two weeks in hospital. The stammer varied and may even have disappeared for some spells, but by the time I reached nine years old it had returned permanently, with sufficient severity for speech therapy to be given. This therapy, of the relaxation type, did not appear to reduce the stammering, which may have been due to my own outlook on stammering at that age. The therapy was stopped when I changed schools at ten and a half years and was restarted at the age of twelve. The therapy was of the same type but with a different therapist; it again had no success and was stopped when I was fifteen.

The stammering continued until I was thirty-four, when I asked my doctor if there were any other forms of therapy available in the area; as a result I went to the Royal Victoria Infirmary in Newcastle.

My stammer at this time consisted of five main parts:
(1) rapid repetition of sounds; (2) prolongations of sounds; (3) total blockages; (4) stammering on an in-breath, and (5) a lot of 'back' noise from my throat.

I did switch words a little and also used adjectives in front of difficult sounds to assist in starting the word. I was not aware that I stammered as much as I did. The severity of the stammer varied and was greatly affected by the situation, e.g. talking to strangers, and also by my health and my emotional state.

At the initial interview with the therapist, easy-stammering was explained to me and a course of treatment was begun (June).

Results were found encouraging as the easy-stammer system was introduced into conversation at home. However, following an enforced break in practice due to vacation and business the progress that had been made was lost.

Progress from the middle of August was good and by early September conversation at home was free from stammering – all stammers were being controlled (80 per cent with good control, 20 per cent with a form of control). This improvement was only with the family and even when friends called the ability to control was greatly reduced.

The problems of control on the 20 per cent with a form of control were found to be on five main sounds, 'm', 'l', 'w', 'y', and 'n', with some occasional difficulty on 'f', 'r', and 's'. Theoretical explanation of the way to handle these sounds, plus easy-stammer reading practice on them for two weeks, improved the control and enabled the majority of 'm's, 'l's, and 'w's to be picked out in advance, allowing an easy-stammer to be inserted even if it was not necessary.

By mid September the easy-stammer had been tried with friends and a reasonable control achieved. It was then decided to try it out in various situations at work. To achieve this, a list of all the situations which occur at work, in their order of severity, was made.

The three easiest situations were handled with little problem and I am now currently (November) trying to control in the first of the hard situations.

The degree of success I can achieve in controlling my stammer depends on the amount of concentration I can employ at that time. It is also very dependent on the situation I am in – being good in one situation does not give any carry over into a different one. Practice of easy-stammering by faking during reading helps and should be carried on as long as possible. Slowing down of talking speed also helps my ability to control – it is easier to concentrate on two things at a time if you are doing them more slowly.

Anything which lessens my power of concentration – e.g. illness, alcohol, tiredness, emotional stress, pressure of work – reduces the amount of control I can achieve.

As my knowledge and use of easy-stammering is increasing I am more aware of stammering (without control) but it is not as severe as that experienced before June; I no longer experience total blocks, nor do I talk on an in-breath. The noise from my throat is also much reduced and it is now just a matter of time, practice and concentration before I can expect to achieve a better overall control of my stammer.

Speak for Yourself · 125

My outlook on life has changed and will change again as my ability to control improves. I feel more at ease at home, with friends, and at work, knowing that I can control my speech to a reasonable standard.

11. MR R.S. (AGE: THIRTY-FOUR)
Description of my stammer before I started speech therapy

1. Frequent use of word avoidances, use of well-worn phrases that contain only words I can say; dentistry is ideal for this as short commands are all that are required most of the time. The avoidances and phrases have been used on and off for twenty years and so are probably ingrained as part of the speaking pattern.
2. Control on problem words by deliberately stopping, gaining relaxation, and then carrying on. Seventy-five per cent of problem words can be dealt with like this, the remaining 25 per cent persisted as definite blocks, e.g. sedative, Robert, three. These problem words can occasionally be said quite fluently depending on circumstances.

    Ways I had of getting round an anticipated blockage (other than above):
    (a) try to use different words to say the same thing,
    (b) use a synonym,
    (c) put an easily sayable word in front of the problem word.
3. Telephone used only when I could not avoid it, never completely happy.
4. Stammer appeared to get worse in conditions of stress, strain, illness, and tiredness; also when having a casual conversation with friends when several speakers contribute rapidly to the conversation.
5. Things that temporarily improved the stammer:
    (a) public speaking,
    (b) speaking in front of strangers and children,
    (c) hearing another person stammering.
6. Stammer appeared to deteriorate over the last two years: became depressed and demoralized over this; for the first

time ever had problems in dentist/patient communication, 'retreated into shell', and only spoke when had to; stammering definitely gets worse towards the end of a working day.

Analysis of stammer

1. Blocks; approach of potential blockages can usually be anticipated.
2. Multiple small stammers, usually in first three or four words of sentence, come and go before being noticed; some are probably never noticed.
3. General rate of speaking too fast.

What has helped me, four months after starting therapy

1. Discussions with speech therapist, and awareness of the problem being tackled, have produced a better mental outlook, i.e. do not now get depressed or demoralized by stammers.
2. Ability to apply easy-stammer in over 75 per cent of potential blockages; easy-stammers appear to go unnoticed – nobody has ever reacted to them by remarks or by facial expression.
3. General slowing down of rate of speaking with particular attention to first three or four words of any sentence. When consciously stop to speak more slowly, the small stammers are virtually non-existent; now managing to do this about 90 per cent of the time.
4. Improvement in confidence generally.

Outlook for the future

1. Fewer stammers make more confidence; already becoming more adventurous in speaking, would help if I intentionally used the 'phone more often.
2. Will continue to concentrate on slowing down of rate of speaking.
3. As the time goes by, easy-stammer is applied more easily, sometimes I find myself using the easy-stammer without consciously applying it.

4. Most of my speaking difficulties are related to any build-up of nervous tension, so attempt to slow down pace of life in general and live and work at a more relaxed pace.

Note: being a dentist gives very good opportunity for what advised to practise.

12. MR V.S. (AGE: FORTY-FIVE)

Before I went for speech therapy, I had a severe stammer; at times it took me at least thirty seconds before I could get a word out, and I used to get a pain in my chest with all the tension. Every time I had to speak to people, friends as well as strangers, I used to panic and sweat a great deal; I couldn't get my words out at all. I very rarely used the telephone as the tension came, and I used to stammer very badly.

When I went to the speech therapist for my first lesson, I can recall I couldn't give my name and address as my stammer was that severe, and I had to write it down on paper.

It took me quite a while to get into the way of easy-stammer, as you have to concentrate very hard, but I find it much more easy now.

I find after I have been for my lesson on a Wednesday, I can go for about five days talking very well with the easy-stammer, and then I seem to lose the concentration till I go back for my next lesson.

At home now I can have a good conversation with my wife, speaking slow, never getting into a fluster, and most of all no tension; a thing I could never do before I took up speech therapy. Easy-stammering has changed my attitude to my stammer, as I don't think about it very much now, and it was always on my mind before.

13. MR K.W. (AGE: TWENTY)

For as long as I can remember, I've always had a stammer, which has been quite severe at times. I remember many a time opening my mouth to make some earth-shattering announcement, or make some witty remark, when I've been just unable to speak, or make any sort of sound, but have just stood, my mouth wide open, and my face rapidly turning crimson in embarrassment. This used always to happen when I was giving someone my name. Gradually, I was able to hide my embarrassment, and just shrug it off. I developed a habit of pulling my hair and rubbing it, with my fingers, against my upper lip, then, if I tried to speak and couldn't, it looked (I thought) as if I had merely opened my mouth to chew my hair. Also, I was always afraid to speak directly at a person, and a habit of rapidly blinking as I spoke developed. At my worst, as I spoke 'to' someone I spoke to my feet, pulled at my hair, and blinked with both eyes.

I've had three unsuccessful attempts to beat my stammer; firstly, up to the age of five years, I attended a reading class held by a local headmistress. This didn't seem to help.

Secondly, I attended therapy in which patients were made to relax by lying on mattresses, pillows, etc. In this relaxed state, patients talked with, or read to, the therapists. This didn't help me, but I feel if I'd been a little older and more urgent it may have helped.

Thirdly, I tried syllable-based speech, which is speaking to a constant rhythm by breaking up each word into syllables. This did not help me at all. I was always afraid to use it outside the clinic because it made speech sound very jerky, and artificial.

By this time, I was about thirteen years old, and I had stopped trying to find a 'cure'. My speech then improved gradually over the next five years, until, at eighteen years of age, I was reasonably efficient, with the help of various 'tricks' like speaking quietly and rapidly, so people would not hear me in full, and word switching. I was always wary of beginning a conversation with a plosive sound, and would switch to a word that was easier to say.

At nineteen I moved from home into a flat, where I lived with two friends. I lived there for ten weeks only, but in this time, for no reason apparent to me, my speech deteriorated until I had lost all confidence, and began to be afraid to ask for bus fares, or go to dentists' or doctors' surgeries, etc. It was at this time that I attended the R.V.I. for speech therapy.

Immediately, I was told that I must slow my speech considerably. I found that by slowing down, my speech improved quite a lot. I found that I stammered a lot less. The easy-stammer ensures that when I do stammer, I can stop, and immediately say the word perfectly, without any periods of embarrassing silence, accompanied by hair pulling, etc. Now, I find that I can always start a conversation easily, and even giving my name to doctors' and dentists' receptionists presents no problem, even over the telephone, which I could never previously do. I find one thing strange though; although my speech is fluent in nearly every situation, it is useless in the clinic! I think this is caused by the people in the group expecting me to stammer, which they obviously do, whereas, outside the clinic, people don't expect it, and I don't think of it before I speak. Anyway, this is only a minor part of my life. I realized years ago that I could never beat my stammer altogether, as it was, and still is, part of me, but I am now sure of controlling it. I am now armed against it.

Children and young people of sixteen years or under

14. A.A. (BOY; AGE: EIGHT)

Two and a half years ago I began to take my son for speech therapy to correct a stammer and for sound defects. The sounds, all except the 'r', are perfect; the stammer has improved a lot but still occurs occasionally. When the stammer does occur, he is learning to control it.

Over the past fifteen months he has had quite a lot of practice in 'elastic' reading; this is stretching the first word of every line he reads. After doing this for about a year we noticed, on one occasion, that he started to say something with difficulty, but he stopped speaking and re-started successfully with an 'elastic' word; after this first word was said, the rest came easily. Since then he has done it quite a lot. Also, he no longer puts his hand over his mouth when he speaks.

Since the first several months of speech therapy my son has not needed to go very often, and he now goes once every three months. He is only eight years old so we hope that he will get over his stammer altogether in time.

15. R.A. (GIRL; AGE: THIRTEEN)

I have been stammering for ten years, starting when I was three years old. At my first primary school I suffered many embarrassing experiences while I was reading. People made fun of me and everyone thought I was queer and left me alone, so I was scared of reading and reciting aloud and I began to cry, usually after two or three words.

I had years of syllable-timed-speech but my stammer only got worse as I grew older, so by the time I went to the R.V.I. I had a very severe stammer with blocks, repetitions, and facial grimaces. I threw back my head and stammered hard, and often covered my mouth with my hand. I did not like the method of therapy I had been taught, so I was only too glad of a change.

After a few weeks of work I could easy-stammer about 50 per cent of the time, both in reading and talking, in the clinic. One night I amazed my mother by reading fluently to her aloud. Later, she said in the clinic, 'It is the first time she has ever been able to read.' Here, at last, was a victory I could triumph over – a transformation from stammering two or three words then bursting into tears! I then began to make steady progress, gradually building up a fortress where I could fight from, to win over the stammer.

I am only unsuccessful when I am in a hurry or am not concentrating very hard. It *is* hard to concentrate all the time but, when I do, my easy-stammer is very good (at least that is what everyone tells me!).

I have been going to the clinic for just over a year – first weekly then fortnightly, and I am going to continue my therapy until I'm almost perfect.

I now know that my stammer is about 75 per cent less frequent and that it is about 85 per cent less tense. When I stammered, my worst situations were school, and when I was out shopping. Now I feel that I am *much* better at both situations and I am *much* happier. If people make fun of me, I am determined to show them what I can really do, so that they are the ones who feel stupid instead of me.

I am often chosen to read in lessons and I have taken one of the leading parts in a form play.

What easy-stammering means to me is hard to say – it means such a lot – but one way of saying it is this: the easy-stammer is a weapon, a sword or spear that I can take up to fight with. Before I had nothing – now I have a weapon which will never fail me – I'll beat the stammer with it yet! In the future I'll expect to have won so many battles against the stammer that I'll be master. I'll expect to have a small 'rebellion' now and then but the stammer will never get the upper hand again, and if it does – it will be my own fault, for not trying to control.

16. L.C. (BOY; AGE: SIXTEEN)

When I first went to therapy I had a severe stammer. My main concern was speaking on stage (I'm in a musical group) which I couldn't do because of my stammer. Also at school I found it difficult; people would make jokes about my speech.

Apart from stammering I spoke very fast; I was told over 200 words a minute.

After a few months using easy-stammering, I lost most of my stammer; my smaller stammer meant I could speak on stage without any trouble. I had to slow down my speech to talk well but if I talked very quickly the stammer returned.

Easy-stammering has now cut out most of my stammer and I can control what is left if I don't talk too quickly; I can speak without stammering, using easy-stammering. This has enabled me to obtain a compère's job in a working-man's club.

Most of my stammer has gone, about 90 per cent. The remainder is not affecting me much because in any situations now I have no trouble with my speech. I can speak to people without the stammer being noticed.

17. J.H. (BOY; AGE: EIGHT)

[This little boy attended for regular weekly speech therapy for less than three months, between the ages of six and a half and six and three quarter years.]

My son's stammer appeared to occur mostly at times of stress or excitement. Before therapy began, his speech under extreme conditions could be almost incoherent. The degree of speech distortion appeared to be correlated with the amount of stress undergone.

However, as treatment progressed, the benefits became more apparent and lasting. Under stress conditions, when words were tumbling one over another, a gentle reminder of 'easy way' produced an immediate improvement, although a reminder was occasionally necessary after the initial check.

As time went by, the necessity for reminders became less frequent, and now only very occasional checks are necessary as my son has learned to control his speech. There is every indication that the treatment has given impressive and lasting results.

18. S.K. (BOY; AGE: FOURTEEN)

When I first attended speech therapy my stammer was very noticeable; I had been stammering for as long as I could remember. But even worse than the stammer was a very severe head jerk. After attending speech therapy and learning to easy-stammer, I found my head jerk disappeared altogether after a few months. I still attend the clinic every few weeks but I have found I am able to cope a lot better with my school work and with my social life since learning easy-stammering.

I think my stammer is about 90 per cent better; I am still working on what's left.

19. P.MCN. (BOY; AGE: FOURTEEN)

When I first started speech therapy, quite a while ago, I had a really bad stammer and could not control it. Also I blocked my words and switched them around so I could say them.

Then I started on easy-stammer; at this time there were words I could not say, like my brother's name. I picked up the habit of using easy-stammer really quickly, and after a few ups and downs I had really improved. Even I thought so. Easy-stammer gave me self-confidence to talk to people, shout, sing, or just read aloud which I could not do before easy-stammer. I think it is revolutionary for people who stammer; pity someone didn't think of it years ago. Really excellent.

20. M.S. (BOY; AGE: FOURTEEN)

I am just fourteen years of age and I have had a stammer since I was four. So far I have only been for speech therapy three times because I am away at boarding school.

My stammer has troubled me most when I am at school and I have to ask or answer questions in class, and when I first went away to school some of the boys laughed at me when I couldn't get my words out.

On my first visit to the speech therapist I was taught how to easy-stammer and since then I have found it easier to ask questions at school, and my stammer has improved by at least 50 per cent. I am also in a smaller form now and the boys who used to laugh at me have gone into a different form and I think this has also helped me to gain more confidence in myself.

I also had trouble with my stammer when asking for anything in shops, but since visiting the speech therapist my mother has noticed that I haven't stammered at all in the shops when I am at home on holiday.

21. D.S. (BOY; AGE: THIRTEEN)

My son had a slight stammer from starting school or maybe it was at the age of six years. Over the next six years his speech slowly became worse until it reached the stage of him having difficulty with general conversation, and great embarrassment when being asked to read in front of the class at school. From about the age of eleven he seemed to 'hibernate' into his room a great deal to listen to records or play games on his own. We have since realized that this was in fact a way out of making conversation with either family or visitors.

On his first visit to the speech therapy unit he could hardly get one word of a paragraph out at all, and this even surprised me, as I had not realized his speech was so bad with strangers. I also fully realized then the embarrassment he must in fact have been suffering.

On writing this, my son has been attending for therapy exactly four months. He has worked very hard at all he has been instructed to do and the result has been tremendous. He is a changed boy, and now goes into company and makes a conversation with anyone he comes into contact with. We have been really amazed at the change in him, and he has lost virtually all his stammer in every speaking situation, and is now quite proud to read out aloud to anyone who asks him.

Recently discharged

22. MR P.C. (AGE: NINETEEN)

When I first went for therapy my speech was very often unintelligible, due to speaking rapidly and to my tense repetitions of sounds and words. My stammer was so bad that when possible I would not use a phone (I work in an office), and unless someone spoke to me I would try to avoid any sort of conversation. This put a great strain on me in and out of work.

On entering therapy I was first told to slow my speech down and then went on to easy-stammering; the result within only two months was fantastic. Everyone I knew commented on my improvement. Even phone calls became less of a physical strain to me; my improvement in that short time alone was near a 100 per cent compared with what it was.

After four months of therapy I was almost stammer-free, and it was not long after this that I found I was actually starting conversations with people! I won't say my stammer has gone completely but I know if a stammer does slip through I will be able to control it.

My friends and family were a great help to me, for I found it very hard to slow my speech down; I had to think about this every hour of the day. For those people who have the same problem as me I cannot stress enough the importance of slowing down your speech, for without this easy-stammering is impossible.

Easy-stammering opened a new life to me; the simple thing of being able to speak when spoken to.

23. MRS B.L. (AGE: THIRTY-THREE)

I would say that the use of easy-stammer has helped tremendously in overcoming my stammer. Although in my case the stammer was not severe, it was still an embarrassment to me, and affected my life in many ways.

At first I had to make a conscious effort to use the easy-stammer but, as time went on, and with more practice, I found I was using it almost without realizing. Only when I had to cope with a really 'sticky' word, did I have to think about it. A general slowing-down of my speech was also very helpful, as the easy-stammer went unnoticed.

Before I used easy-stammer, I would never dare to speak out in a group of people, although there were lots of things I would have liked to say. But before I could speak, there would be a tightness in my throat, my hands would go clammy, and my heart would start to race. As a result, I became too tense to say anything, knowing that I would be unable to speak without stammering. Once I had got used to the easy-stammer, however, I was able to control the stammer to such an extent that the tension disappeared, and now I no longer worry so much about speaking in a crowd. There is still the occasional moment when the stammer comes through, but this does not worry me nearly as much as it used to, as I realize now that even non-stammerers are apt to trip over words occasionally.

I am still not very keen on the telephone, although I answer when it rings with no difficulty. Only on out-going calls do I still feel a slight panic beforehand, but nothing like as bad as it used to be, and I usually find that I make the call with no difficulty. Before I used easy-stammer, I would avoid making calls whenever I possibly could, to the extent that I would drag myself to the doctor, rather than phone and ask him to call.

There are still times when the stammer comes through, despite easy-stammer, but this is due to outside influences, and not to the fear of the stammer itself. Tiredness or illness also make a difference, and make the stammer more difficult to control, but as I know that these things are only temporary, I am not too concerned about it.

I don't know whether I could accurately put the improvement in my speech into figures, but I would say of the stammer which now remains that about 20 per cent occurs at times of particular stress when I am not able to control it as well as I would like; the other 80 per cent of the time I am able to control the stammer completely.

24. MISS E.T. (AGE: TWENTY-TWO) (discharged on leaving the district)

The problem of my particular stammer was being asked direct questions; the stammer was not greatly in evidence until someone asked me a direct question, when I would start to stammer badly. I have always had a problem like telling someone my name and address, which is a singularly embarrassing one. I remember the nearest description I have heard of my sort of stammer, particularly on these occasions, is a 'machine-gun in the larynx'.

Easy-stammering helped me in these situations because I learned not to panic or get wound up when a direct question was fired at me, but just to take my time answering it. Easy-stammering has also been a help as like many people who stammer, I suppose, I tend to talk quickly to get it over with in a hurry. Talking quickly, I have found, definitely causes more stammers, most of them through carelessness, but easy-stammering tends to slow you down and make you more careful.

I think the reason easy-stammering has helped me is because it is the most practical method I have used, and it sounds the most natural with practice. Going to the clinic group, also, was very helpful because it gave us all a chance to talk over our problems, and it gave me the somewhat daunting experience (at first) of hearing what other people who stammer sound like. It was very good for me because I realized that my problem, compared with other people's at the clinic, was not as bad as I had thought, and it made me see it in proportion. It was comforting to hear other people talk about problems which I had previously believed exclusive to me; for example, I was very relieved to hear that I was not the only person who hated using the phone in case an awkward or direct question was asked.

I doubt if there will ever be a miracle cure for stammering, but I think that easy-stammering cuts the problem down to size and provides a practical method of controlling the stammer.

25. MR G.W. (AGE: FORTY-ONE)

When I was five years old I witnessed a serious explosion in which several people were killed; it was after this that my nerves were affected and an impediment in my speech started. At school I had great difficulty in reading in class without kicking my leg; even then it would probably take me twenty to thirty seconds to get started. I would not do errands for my mother. I found it practically impossible to ask for fares on a bus unless I had the correct change in my hand.

I improved over the years, replacing kicking with clenched fists, but I still had great difficulty in reading in public, asking for fares, or directions. I never used the telephone and would not enter into discussions unless with close friends. I would switch words and even re-phrase a sentence after being half way through it.

When I was forty years old I sought the advice of my doctor who made an appointment for me at the R.V.I. speech therapy unit, where the therapist explained the easy-stammer method of speech control.

This method has helped me immensely. I am no longer tensed up (i.e. clenching my fist); it has slowed my speech down, as talking quickly is one of the downfalls of a person who stammers. Even after a frustrating day's driving I find by using the easy-stammer I can talk to people quite well.

As I said, previously I would not even enter into a discussion and yet, after only nine visits to the unit, I addressed a meeting of 160 people for three to four minutes; I made my point, introduced a touch of successful humour, and summed up – without one hesitation. I was even congratulated later on my speech. I will be eternally grateful for the easy-stammer method of speech control.

Suggestions for Study

In keeping with the simple and practical nature of this book, I have only touched briefly upon the concepts, theories, and therapies of stammering. It may well be that some readers will wish to explore further into the details of the problem and I am therefore including a book list of suggested reading.

Andrews, G., and Harris, M., *The Syndrome of Stuttering*, London, The Spastics Society Medical Education and Information Unit, in association with Heinemann, 1964.

Bloodstein, O., *A Handbook on Stuttering*, Chicago National Easter Seal Society for Crippled Children and Adults, 1969.

Hahn, F. H., *Stuttering, Significant Theories and Therapies*, 2nd ed. prepared by E. S. Hahn, 4th printing, Stanford, California, Stanford University Press, 1968.

Hunt, J., *Stammering and Stuttering, Their Nature and Treatment*, orginally published 1861; reprint: introduction by E. J. Schaffer, New York, Hafner, 1967.

Johnson, W., et al., *Speech Handicapped School Children*, 3rd ed., New York, Harper & Row, 1967.

Muirden, R., *Stammering – Its Correction Through the Re-education of the Speech Function*, Springfield, Illinois, Charles C. Thomas, 1968.

Schwartz, M. F., *Stuttering Solved*, London, Heinemann, 1976.

Van Riper, C., *The Nature of Stuttering*, Englewood Cliffs, New Jersey, Prentice-Hall, 1971.

Van Riper, C., *The Treatment of Stuttering*, Englewood Cliffs, New Jersey, Prentice-Hall, 1973.

Wohl, Maud T., 'The Electronic Metronome – An Evaluative Study', *British Journal of Disorders of Communications*, 3, 1, pp. 89–98, 1968.

More About Penguins and Pelicans

Penguinews, which appears every month, contains details of all the new books issued by Penguins as they are published. It is supplemented by our stocklist, which includes almost 5,000 titles.

A specimen copy of *Penguinews* will be sent to you free on request. Please write to Dept EP, Penguin Books Ltd, Harmondsworth, Middlesex, for your copy.

In the U.S.A.: For a complete list of books available from Penguins in the United States write to Dept CS, Penguin Books, 625 Madison Avenue, New York, New York 10022.

In Canada: For a complete list of books available from Penguins in Canada write to Penguin Books Canada Ltd, 2801 John Street, Markham, Ontario L3R 1B4.

In Australia: For a complete list of books published by Penguins in Australia write to the Marketing Department, Penguin Books Australia Ltd, P.O. Box 257, Ringwood, Victoria 3134.

Recent Books on Health and Medicine in Penguins

Health Rights Handbook
A Guide to Medical Care
Gerry and Carol Stimson

A completely up-to-date guide to the medical facilities available to you in Britain. The authors believe that *your body belongs to you and only you should decide what to do with it and what to have done to it*. Their book will help you to understand the NHS itself and to deal with doctors and other health workers in order to get the most out the services available.

Our Bodies Ourselves
A Health Book by and for women
Boston Women's Health Book Collective
British Edition by *Angela Phillips and Jill Rakusen*

The most successful book about women ever published, *Our Bodies Ourselves* has sold over one million copies worldwide.
'Every woman in the country should be issued with a copy free of charge' – *Mother and Baby*
'Well researched, informative and educational for both men and women' – *British Medical Journal*
'The Bible of the woman's health movement' – *Guardian*
'If there's only one book you ever buy – this should be it' – *19*

The NHS: Your Money or Your Life
Lesley Garner

We all recognise the symptoms – growing waiting lists, inadequate facilities particularly for the elderly and the handicapped, dissatisfied doctors, strained industrial relations – but precisely what is the NHS disease? In this comprehensive study, Lesley Garner analyses the problems, and argues for a radical change in social attitudes, which would incorporate a re-examination of the 1946 NHS Act.

Treat Yourself to Sex
A Guide to Good Loving
Paul Brown and Carolyn Faulder

'We are writing for people who may, or may not, be highly experienced sexually and who, for reasons beyond their comprehension, find that sex is not the pleasure that they would like.'

Basic, readable, sympathetic, this handbook deals with a range of sexual problems that are more common than generally supposed, and gives a series of exercises, 'sexpieces', worked out after extensive research, which, if followed honestly and carefully, will help provide workable solutions.

Boy Girl Man Woman
A Guide to Sex for Young People
B. H. Claësson

Here at last is a book devoted to the special needs of the young. Informative and sympathetic, it enables them to increase their sexual awareness and enjoy their own sexuality.

'*Boy Girl Man Woman* is excellent. It provides clarity and humanity in just the right mixture. Adolescents will find it immensely helpful and reassuring' – James Hemming

The Body
Anthony Smith

Anthony Smith examines, with rare individuality, the human body, its functions, its abilities and its peculiarities. Sex and reproduction, being the mainstay of the life-cycle, form his central theme; this is supplemented by an unexpected variety of information about such things as inheritance, circumcision, haemophilia, twinning, and many other topics seldom explored or explained.

Later chapters deal with other bodily functions, such as the senses, digestion, sleep, and the skeleton, all accompanied by relevant, curious facts, which make the subject all the more fascinating.

Penguins for Parents

The Myth of the Hyperactive Child
And Other Means of Child Control
Peter Schrag and Diane Divoky

'A well-researched and thoughtfully argued brief intended to stimulate action against the widespread use of drugs, psychological testing, and behaviour modification used by agents of the state to control children's lives and undermine their rights' – *The New York Times Book Review*

The Special Child
The Education of Mentally Handicapped Children
Barbara Furneaux

Written to help and to evaluate the help that is available for mentally handicapped children. Here Barbara Furneaux argues for a more caring and supportive attitude on the part of society, and for a greater financial commitment to the handicapped child, as she believes that, with sufficient individual attention, even the severely handicapped child is educable.

Helping Your Handicapped Child
A Step-by-Step Guide to Everyday Problems
Janet Carr

'Anyone who has to cope day by day with a handicapped child will benefit from this book' – Elizabeth Newson

Your Child's Teeth
A Parent's Guide to Making and Keeping them Perfect
Stephen J. Moss

Bad teeth don't 'run in the family'. There is no hereditary excuse for cavities or for crooked teeth. Instead, children acquire from us early habits, muscular patterns, attitudes to oral cleanliness and so forth. With Stephen Moss's book we can ensure they acquire *good* habits.

Children Growing Up
Eurfron Gwynne Jones

By taking a camera into ordinary homes Dr Eurfron Gwynne Jones was able to build up a detailed record of a young child over a period of time. Here she describes and assesses children – at first with their mothers, and then discovering the world, reacting to strangers and learning to walk, talk and play.

'Children do not just grow – they are "brought up",' she concludes. The love and encouragement of their parents (or those who care for them) are the most important things in their lives. An unloved, unwanted child has little chance of becoming a happy, healthy adult.

Play With a Purpose for Under Sevens
E. M. Matterson

In this new edition of *Play With a Purpose for Under Sevens* the author gathers together information about pre-school playgroups which has emerged in the last decade (information obtained from watching, talking and working with mothers and young children) and suggests answers to some of the questions which have arisen.

Elizabeth Matterson includes chapters on natural play materials, providing for physical activity and imaginative play. As she herself says in the last chapter 'Children's early years are vitally important and they need plenty of things and people to play with.'

Help Your Child to Read and Write, and More
David Mackay and Joseph Simo

This handbook is not intended as a substitute for professional teaching in schools, but as a preparation for it. With clear and copious illustrations the authors show how parents can provide the right environment for reading and writing at home. They show how to make picture books; how handwriting can grow out of painting; how to recognize and relate different sounds, letters and words. They also give full information about books to look at and read with young children.